Children's Hospices:
A lifeline for families?

Carol Robinson and Pat Jackson

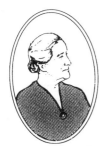

SUPPORTED BY

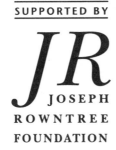

JR
JOSEPH
ROWNTREE
FOUNDATION

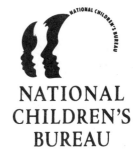

NATIONAL
CHILDREN'S
BUREAU

The National Children's Bureau (NCB) works to identify and promote the well-being and interests of all children and young people across every aspect of their lives.

It encourages professionals and policy makers to see the needs of the whole child and emphasises the importance of multidisciplinary, cross-agency partnerships. The NCB has adopted and works within the UN Convention on the Rights of the Child.

It collects and disseminates information about children and promotes good practice in children's services through research, policy and practice development, membership, publications, conferences, training and an extensive library and information service.

Several Councils and Fora are based at the NCB and contribute significantly to the breadth of its influence. It also works in partnership with Children in Scotland and Children in Wales and other voluntary organisations concerned for children and their families.

The **Joseph Rowntree Foundation** has supported this project as part of its programme of research and innovative development projects, which it hopes will be of value to policy makers and practitioners.

The views expressed in this book are those of the author and not necessarily those of the National Children's Bureau or the Joseph Rowntree Foundation.

Published by National Children's Bureau Enterprises Ltd, 8 Wakley Street, London EC1V 7QE

National Children's Bureau Enterprises Ltd is the trading company for the National Children's Bureau (Registered Charity number 258825).

Typeset by LaserScript Ltd, Mitcham, Surrey CR4 4NA

Printed and bound in the United Kingdom by Redwood Books, Trowbridge BA14 8RN

Contents

List of tables

Acknowledgements

This book is based on the work of four children's hospices and without the help of hospice staff, we could not have undertaken our research. Not only did they provide us with direct assistance with the data collection but also a great deal of friendliness and hospitality. We are most grateful to them for all the time and energy they put into the project. We are also highly indebted to the families we interviewed for giving up their precious time and for sharing their experiences so willingly.

During the fieldwork, we were fortunate to have the assistance of Sheila Body, Paul Brady, Julia Mansfield, Beth Neill and Zoë Taylor. Thanks go to them for their support and interest. We are also grateful to Maggie Barker, Claire Benjamin, Lesley Campbell, Hazel Curtis, Mary Lewis, Trisha Nash, Maureen Oswin, Linda Ward, and Keith Young for their advice and comments on the research questions and findings.

Alison Wertheimer has edited the final report with great care and we are especially grateful to her for her hard work and patience. We also wish to thank Jane Charlton for her conscientious secretarial support throughout the project. Finally, our thanks go to the Joseph Rowntree Foundation for their support, which enabled us to undertake this study.

About the authors

Carol Robinson

Carol Robinson (BA Hons, CQSW, Dip ASS, PhD) is a Senior Research Fellow and project director at the Norah Fry Research Centre, University of Bristol. Her special interests are the rights of disabled children and adults, and effective support services for families. Prior to coming to the University she was a social worker for Essex County Council. Carol carried out a PhD in the School of Education at Bristol and joined the Department in 1983. She has published articles, pamphlets and books, notably on short-term breaks. A previous NCB book *Balancing the Act*, co-authored with Margaret Macadam, was published in 1995.

Pat Jackson

Pat Jackson (MSc, BA Hons, CQSW) joined the Norah Fry Research Centre in 1996 as a Research Associate to work on the project 'The Role of Children's Hospices in the Provision of Short Term Care'. She started her research career in the Department of Social Medicine (also at the University of Bristol) where she worked on studies looking at palliative care provision for adults both within community and hospice settings. In addition she spent a short period of time working with the Health Promotion Research Programme on a range of projects including accident prevention in schools, smoking and pregnancy, and back pain in nurses. Pat has experience as a practitioner of working with disabled people in both hospital and community-based settings. Her research interests include palliative care provision and the health/social care interface of service provision for both children and adults.

Summary of findings

The study

The study was concerned with short-term care arrangements in children's hospices between 1996 and 1998 and was supported by the Joseph Rowntree Foundation. The research looked at: which children are using hospices; why families use this service; what kind of care children receive at the hospice, the families' views and experiences; and how hospices are regulated. Four children's hospices participated in the study which involved records searches; interviews with families, external professionals and hospice staff, and observations at each site.

The children

- 358 children had stayed at the hospices in one year.
- The average age was 9.7 years and nearly two thirds were males.
- Over half the children had diseases of the nervous system and one third had cerebral palsy.
- A fifth had severely limited life expectancy and just over a half might survive into adulthood.
- Many children required high levels of nursing care but nearly a quarter required none.
- Children using hospice care tended to be younger, to require more nursing care and more often have life-limiting conditions than children using other short-term care services.

The families

- Almost a third were lone parent families.
- A quarter of fathers were unemployed.
- Twelve per cent of families were from minority ethnic communities.

- Families appreciated hospice care because of: the non-clinical environment; good facilities and quality of care; the friendliness of staff; and the breaks from caring.
- Parents' few complaints included: distance from home; having to transport the child's equipment; and insufficient breaks, especially during weekends and school holidays.
- Only a minority of families had ever had meetings with hospice staff to discuss their child's care.

Use of other services

- Over a third of families had never used any other short-term care services.
- Nearly two thirds were using at least one other service (family link, sitting services, holiday playschemes).
- Most families had been offered hospital-based care but few had used it and families were often not happy with it.
- Some children using hospices were not eligible for local services because of their needs and level of disability.

Eligibility criteria

- There were no uniform eligibility criteria across the hospices.
- Newer hospices often have looser criteria than more established ones which tend to only provide for children with life-limiting conditions.
- A quarter of all referrals were made by medical practitioners, just over a fifth by social workers, a quarter from other professionals and the remainder from the families themselves.
- Professionals were concerned about the more restrictive eligibility criteria in some hospices and the lack of provision for young adults.

Use of hospice care

- Families used hospice care because of: positive recommendations, unsatisfactory experiences elsewhere and a lack of suitable alternatives.
- Nearly four fifths of admissions were for short-term care, the remainder being emergency admissions.

- Average number of stays per year was seven; nearly a third had fewer than four stays; nearly one in 20 children were admitted more than once a month.
- On average, children stayed 20 days a year.

The children's experiences

- Most children appeared to enjoy their hospice stays, a view endorsed by most parents.
- However, nearly half the families mentioned changes in their child after a hospice stay which seemed to indicate homesickness.
- A lack of planned activities and stimulation was observed, particularly for children with severe or multiple impairments.
- The mix of ages, and frail children with more active children, could pose potential risks at times.

Staff and volunteers

- The proportion of trained nurses varied but there was always at least one on duty at any one time.
- The ratio of trained to untrained staff also varied, although parents and some professionals thought that all care staff were qualified nurses.
- Hospices did not always have effective mechanisms for bringing in extra personnel at short notice so staff were sometimes working under a lot of pressure.
- Some staff worked very long hours without proper breaks.
- Teamwork was generally good, although it could be hard to maintain at times.
- Volunteers were involved in a range of tasks including practical work as well as direct work with children and families in some cases.
- Some hospices had independent counsellors to support staff and volunteers, although they were not always used.

Professionals and the hospices

- Most considered that hospice care was superior to other short-term services.
- Some professionals had good working relationships with hospice staff but others received little information,

making it difficult for them to work effectively with
families.

Regulation

- Children's hospices are registered as nursing homes which
  many hospice managers thought unsatisfactory.
- The outreach services developed by some hospices are not
  subject to registration and inspection requirements.
- Children using hospices do not fall within the remit of the
  Arrangements for Placement of Children Regulations
  1991 (Children Act) which means that the placement is
  not subject to formal review.

Case study 1: Jonathan

Jonathan is ten and lives with his mum in a fourth-floor flat on a large council estate. He has cerebral palsy and severe epilepsy. Because he finds it difficult to swallow, he eats very slowly, so for the last 18 months he had been having supplementary feeds through a gastrostomy tube. As a result, Jonathan has put on weight and is more alert.

However, the extra weight means his mum now struggles to carry him upstairs, so she has requested a housing transfer and they hope to be rehoused in a few months' time.

One weekend a month, Jonathan stays with another family, which is organised by social services. This works well but Jonathan's mum needed more help and asked for short-term residential care. However, because of Jonathan's tube feeding this wasn't possible, so the social worker suggested approaching the hospice.

Jonathan was assessed by the hospice and offered one weekend a month, with an annual review. His mum stayed with him the first two visits but a year after starting to use hospice care, he now goes on his own. He seems to settle well when he's there and his mum is grateful for the extra break.

1   Children's hospices

Introduction

This publication is based on a study of the role of hospices as providers of short-term (respite) care for disabled children carried out between January 1996 and December 1997. The project, one of a series on children's short-term care carried out at the Norah Fry Research Centre, was undertaken because of the growing importance of children's hospices in supporting families with sick or disabled children and the dearth of research in this area.

Our research, which was supported by the Joseph Rowntree Foundation, explored the impact of hospice care on: the children and their families, including siblings; the professionals supporting them; and the hospice staff and volunteers. In particular it sought to answer the following questions:

- What are the characteristics and needs of children using hospices?
- Is there any overlap between these children and those using other short-term care facilities such as health units or local authority hostels and could this local provision cater for the children currently using hospices?
- How much care do the children receive and how much time do they spend in hospice care?
- Why do families use hospices and why do professionals refer children to them?
- What kinds of experiences do the children have in hospices?
- What do families think about the service they receive?
- How are hospices regulated?

The report concludes with recommendations for future policy and practice.

Background

The general public's prevalent view of children's hospices is that they are places where children with leukaemias and other cancers go to die (Chadwick, 1993). The reality, though, is somewhat different. Early research (Burne, Baum and Dominica, 1984) at Helen House, the first children's hospice, found that only seven per cent of children had these conditions and only 11 per cent were admitted for terminal care. The majority of admissions were for short-term care to provide parents with a break.

This is confirmed by subsequent research (Thornes, 1990) which found that children's hospices were catering for three groups:

- those with **life-limiting** progressive and degenerative conditions such as muscular dystrophy, cystic fibrosis and the mucopolysaccharidoses;
- those with **life-threatening** diseases such as leukaemia, liver disease or severe heart malformation;
- those with a potentially **life-threatening** handicap (*sic*).

Our research was particularly concerned with the third group identified by Thornes namely those who have severe and profound impairments which require 'nursing care' but whose life expectancy is enhanced by treatment. (Tube-fed children, for example, may enjoy much longer and healthier lives than would have been possible with limited oral feeding.)

Children's hospices have a dual function as providers of both short-term care and palliative or terminal care. However, research has not questioned the appropriateness of this and it was one issue which our research sought to examine.

Hospice care for children is growing fast. By mid-1998, there were 11 children's hospices in the UK, with a further 11 in the pipeline. Yet for over a decade concerns have been voiced about the role of these establishments – concerns which are still relevant today.

At a national conference (Salvage, 1986), concern was expresed about the possible unplanned expansion of children's hospices which might result from enthusiasm for helping dying children rather than in response to a genuine and well researched need for a buildings-based service. This expansion of hospice building would also appear to contradict the view of Dame Cicely Saunders, who founded the hospice movement and set up the first adult hospice in the UK, that 'hospice' was a philosophy rather than a facility.

Others have also questioned whether children's hospices are an appropriate and effective response to the needs of children and young people with life-threatening diseases (Chambers, 1987; Carlisle, 1988; Clarke, 1993b).

There is currently no formal definition of what constitutes a children's hospice and there are no national standards. The Association of Children's Hospices (ACH) is presently drawing up national standards, but not all hospices are members of ACH.

The hospices operate as autonomous bodies with charitable status and, to date, central government has paid minimal attention to their regulation. They are currently treated as nursing homes and despite the fact that they accommodate children are exempt from the Children Act regulations.

The study

The four hospices

The hospices were selected, taking into account the following variables:

- how long the hospice had been in operation;
- geographical location (urban and rural locations);
- ages and numbers of children using the hospice;
- funding base (for example, supported through fundraising or by local health authority/trust).

Four hospices participated in the study (a fifth declining on the grounds that it did not accommodate children who would survive into adulthood). Brief descriptions of them are given below (with names changed). One hospice was new and the others were well established. Their size varied between one accommodating 24 children over a year and another 150, though none had more than ten beds. At the start of the research, only one hospice had negotiated payments from health trusts for individual children and none had block contracts.

Aster House opened in 1995, and caters for 24 children up to four-years-old. The hospice takes referrals from hospitals, nurseries, social workers and family members, and can accommodate up to six children at any one time.

The unit is situated within a large former convent building and there are basic facilities for families to stay. The hospice has an outside play area and is close to local amenities and transport.

Begonia House was set up in 1988 and serves approximately 300 children, many of them referred through the local community support team. It caters for children of all ages and has a significant number of children from minority ethnic groups. The hospice is purpose built and can accommodate ten children. It has self-contained family accommodation within the main building, a hydrotherapy pool, games room, multisensory room and a memorial garden. The hospice is close to local amenities and transport.

Cherry Blossoms is located in a large city and was opened in 1991. It is purpose built, currently provides a service to 140 families and can accommodate seven children at any one time. The hospice has self-contained family accommodation separate from the main building, a hydrotherapy pool, multisensory room and an outdoor play area. There is also a non-denominational chapel in the main building. The hospice is close to local amenities and transport. It is adjacent to a children's charity run by a religious foundation.

Daisy Way, which opened in 1991, is in a rural area and has a large catchment area, some children travelling to it from London. The hospice is in a large converted coach-house in the grounds of a religious order. There is limited family accommodation on the same floor as the children's bedrooms. Daisy Way caters for approximately 90 children and can accommodate six at any one time. Owing to its rural location, public transport and local amenities are more limited than with the other hospices.

Facilities varied between the hospices. Some had single bedrooms for the children, while others provided shared sleeping accommodation. Communal areas also varied, with some having more quiet spaces to which children and/or families could retreat if they wished.

Methodology

In devising a methodology for the study, our aims were to:

- analyse data on all short-term admissions to the hospices and ascertain who was eligible to use the service;

- observe how children spent their time in hospice care;
- consult with parents about their reasons for using hospice care, experiences of the services, and level of satisfaction with the hospice;
- ascertain the reasons professionals referred children to hospices and their views on the care provided.

The following methods were used:

- a record search in each hospice;
- interviews with families, hospice staff and referring professionals;
- observations in the hospices.

Record search

Detailed information was gathered from the hospices on 358 children who had used the service between 1 April 1995 and 31 March 1996. The following data were gathered:

- child's age, gender and ethnic background;
- medical diagnosis;
- reason for admission;
- length of time they had been using the hospice;
- referral source;
- number, length and frequency of admissions;
- range of therapies, drugs and treatments provided.

Interviews

Thirty-eight families were interviewed in their own homes, representing 39 children. The families were selected from amongst the 101 children who had conditions such as cerebral palsy, and brain reduction disorders such as microcephaly where the child was expected to survive beyond childhood.

Seventeen professionals who made referrals to three of the hospices were interviewed. They included:

- health visitors (3);
- social workers (3);
- school nurses (2);
- other paediatric nurses (5);
- others (physiotherapist, teacher, paediatrician, GP).

Observations

One of the researchers and a co-observer spent three days in each hospice, observing children and staff. We had hoped to consult with the children themselves, but given the severity of their impairments this did not prove feasible within the time available. However, there were unstructured conversations with other young people who were in residence during the periods of observation.

Case study 2: Emma

Emma is four and lives with her parents and twelve-year-old twin brothers, Tom and Jess. The family has a spacious detached house on the edge of a large commuter village, the accommodation having been adapted for Emma's needs. Emma's dad works in the nearest city and her mum teaches part-time at a local primary school.

According to Emma's mum, her daughter was okay at birth but became very ill a few days later. For what seemed like a long time, no one seemed to know what was wrong, then the family were told she had a viral infection. Emma spent most of the next two years in hospital and on several occasions was not expected to survive.

The infection has left Emma with severe brain damage, poorly controlled epilepsy and unable to sit up or move without help. Her frequent muscle spasms mean that moving or carrying her can be difficult. Emma is also partially sighted though she reacts quite strongly to changes in light.

Emma's parents were devastated when they realised she was not going to recover and still feel 'sad and angry about this at times'.

Although she does not speak, Emma is able to let you know if she is happy or sad by her facial expressions. As her mum says, 'it's important that those who care for her spend time getting to know her so they can tune in to her way of communicating'. Four days a week while her mother is at work, Emma attends a local nursery and seems to enjoy this.

Just over two years ago, one of Emma's consultants suggested that the children's hospice might be willing to look after Emma. It would, he said, give the family a break and provide a similar level of care to the hospital.

Initially Emma's parents were uncertain, but when they heard they could stay with her and help her settle they agreed. Emma's brothers who, as their mum says, are 'very protective' towards their young sister, were also worried but the whole family is now quite relaxed when Emma goes to the hospice for a few days every six weeks.

At first, Emma's mum stayed with her at the hospice, but Emma now stays on her own, though her brothers have sometimes stayed in the school holidays.

Emma's mum finds it quite difficult to keep her interested and alert when there is just the two of them at home, so when Emma is at the hospice she enjoys the stimulation of being surrounded by other children as well as the physical contact with the staff. She also gets plenty of one-to-one attention at the hospice and gets on well with several of the staff who have got to know her over the past couple of years. Emma's parents feel she misses all this when she returns home and have noticed that she can be 'quite grizzly for a couple of days'.

One of Emma's favourite activities at the hospice is spending time in the multi-sensory room and, according to her mum, she would happily stay there for hours. She also enjoys the occasional music sessions.

The family are reluctant to consider any other short-term care for Emma. They feel it took quite a while before they were confident about letting her be cared for by other people. They also worry that if Emma was unwell 'most places would be reluctant to take her'. The fact that the hospice *will* take her even if she is poorly is important because although her health is somewhat better, she does still pick up infections easily.

The family appreciate the support they get from the hospice. Emma's mum, in particular, feels she gets a lot of moral support from the staff in addition to the extra stimulation Emma gets.

2 Who uses the hospices and how

One of the main reasons for undertaking this research was the lack of existing information about which children are using hospices. The first part of this chapter provides a detailed picture of the children using four hospices. The second part looks at issues relating to access and referral, eligibility criteria and possible barriers to access.

The children

Records from the four hospices indicated that between 1 April 1995 and 31 March 1996, 358 children had stayed overnight or longer.

Age and gender

Of the 358 children:

- the youngest was six months and the oldest over 20 years;
- their average age was nine years, seven months;
- 64 per cent were males and 36 per cent females.

Table A1 in the Appendix gives the average age of the children in each hospice.

There are a number of possible reasons why male children comprise almost two thirds of hospice users. There is in general a higher incidence of boys than girls who have a learning disability. Certain conditions, notably Duchenne muscular dystrophy, are also gender related.

Ethnicity

Not all hospices recorded the ethnic origin of both parents, but we were able to classify the children into five broad groupings

(Table 2.1). Three quarters of the Asian children and all those of 'mixed parentage' were using one hospice.

Table 2.1   The ethnic origins of the children

Broad ethnic group	Number	%
White British	314	87.7
Asian	37	10.3
African-Caribbean	2	0.6
African	1	0.6
Mixed parentage	4	1.0
Total	358	100

Diagnoses/conditions

Children using the hospices tended to have a wide range of life-limiting or life-threatening conditions. This study was particularly interested in children who had a 'handicap (*sic*) which is so severe as to be a threat to life' (Thornes, 1990) but who may survive into adulthood. In order to identify those children, we grouped them by diagnoses and prognosis.

Using the *Manual of International Classification of Diseases and Injuries and Causes of Death* (WHO, 1975), the children were allocated to ten broad groupings, details of which can be found in Table A2 in the Appendix. Seven children had not received a definitive diagnosis and are therefore recorded as 'no diagnosis'.

The most common diagnoses, based on the ICD classification were as follows:

- over 50 per cent had disorders of the nervous system, the most common being cerebral palsy and Duchenne muscular dystrophy;
- nearly 30 per cent of the children had congenital abnormalities, the most common being: conditions related to the brain such as microcephaly, encephaly and hydrocephaly; rare or unspecified abnormalities such as tuberous sclerosis; and chromosomal abnormalities such as Down's syndrome;
- just over seven per cent had endocrinal, nutritional and metabolic disorders such as bilary atresia.

Prognosis

In order to decide who they can help, the hospices have to decide which children have life-limiting or life-threatening conditions. However, even with all the relevant information on a child, deciding on a likely prognosis is not an exact science and children frequently defy all the odds and continue to survive. Furthermore, within each diagnostic grouping there can be a wide range of symptoms and attendant impairments which may significantly affect life expectancy.

We consulted numerous texts on childhood diseases and illnesses (Thompson and O'Quinn, 1979; Rendell-Short, Gray and Dodge (1985); Clayden and Hawkins, 1988; Campbell and McIntosh, 1992; Contact A Family Directory, 1997) and referred specific queries to professionals working in the field. We also took account of the care and treatment regimes of each child. Table 2.2 indicates the number of children under each grouping.

Follow-up of the children suggested that our groupings were fairly sound. At the end of 1996 only 20 of the 187 children we thought *might* survive into adulthood had died and only eight of the 99 who *had* been expected to survive into adulthood. A further 40 deaths had occured, all of children with severely limited life expectancy.

There was some variation between the hospices, one having a higher percentage of children likely to die in childhood.

Table 2.2   Estimated prognosis

Prognosis	Number of children	% of children
Life expectancy severely limited (unlikely to survive beyond childhood)	72	20.1
Prognosis less clear (*may* survive into adulthood depending on a number of factors)	187	52.2
Survival into adulthood	99	27.7
Total	358	100

The children's care needs

Information was gathered on the nursing interventions these children required and the medication they needed.

Nursing interventions

As expected, many children required high levels of nursing care. However, 17 per cent of the young people required no nursing care and in a few cases no personal care of any type. These were often older teenagers with physical impairments caused by degenerative diseases such as muscular dystrophy.

Table A3 in the Appendix provides detailed information on the nursing interventions the children required. There was a wide range of tasks, the most common being:

- administration of drugs (75 per cent);
- feeding via gastrostomy tube (20 per cent) or naso-gastric tube (11 per cent);
- suction (11 per cent);
- administration of enemas or suppositories (11 per cent).

Some nursing tasks were required regularly but others were only needed if the child's condition deteriorated or became unstable. In addition, about one in four children required pain relief and one in six used an inhaler (see Table A4 in the Appendix for further details).

Medication

Table A4 in the Appendix indicates the range of drugs prescribed, the frequency of times cited and the number and percentage of children receiving them. Over three quarters of the children required medication, the vast majority on a daily basis. Some individual children required as many as 18 different types of drugs, although the average was 3.5. The most commonly administered drugs were:

- anti-epileptics (50 per cent of children);
- laxatives (26 per cent).

Hospices and other short-term care

The children using hospices were compared with disabled children using other short-term care facilities, drawing on a study of other forms of short-term care (Robinson and Stalker, 1990) including local authority residential homes and hostels, children's hospital wards and specialist health authority short-term care units.

Age

The average age of the children using hospices was nine years seven months, compared with an average of 15 years 1 month in local authority homes and 14 years 1 month in health facilities (although 34 per cent of this last group were under ten years).

Gender

Hospice users comprised 64 per cent boys and 36 per cent girls, compared with 58 per cent and 42 per cent respectively in other residential facilities.

Ethnic background

Nearly 88 per cent of the hospice children were White British, the other significant grouping being Asian children (ten per cent). White British children comprised 91 per cent of users of local authority residential facilities and 81 per cent of children using health authority short-term care facilities.

Nursing, other care and medication

All the children needed assistance with most aspects of daily living, including eating, toileting and getting around, but the hospice children needed more nursing care, particularly tube feeding and suction. However, as the efficacy of suction has become clearer, it has probably also become more common (Hutchinson (1997), personal communication). With the growth of gastrostomy feeding (Micklewright, 1996), tube feeding is also more frequently used than before.

Diagnoses

Although children with cerebral palsy accounted for 18 per cent of hospice children and 20 per cent of those using other facilities, hospices were catering for young people with muscular dystrophy whereas the other facilities previously studied did not.

Prognosis

Twenty per cent of the hospice children had severely limited life expectancy, compared with only three per cent of the children using other facilities in 1990.

In summary, the hospice children:

- tended to be younger;
- required more nursing interventions;
- included a higher percentage who were not expected to reach adulthood.

Access and referral to hospice care

Eligibility criteria

The Guidelines of the Association of Children's Hospices (ACH, 1995) state that:

> the service offered by a children's hospice will be available to children and adolescents with a life-limiting condition and their families.

By using the term 'life-limiting', the Guidelines suggest that admission criteria hinge upon the nature of the child's condition and assessed life expectancy. This was reflected by one of the professionals we interviewed, who commented: 'We are having problems with children who do not fit the criteria for hospice care.'

However, as children's hospices have become more widely known and thus oversubscribed, they have had to apply increasingly stringent eligibility criteria. One of the four hospices in our study had developed a scoring system and another two use a panel of relevant professionals to decide who will receive a service. Only the most recently-opened hospice does not yet have to apply such a formal approach to decision making and can accept families who say they need hospice care for their child.

Some referring professionals expressed concern that these more restrictive entry criteria meant that some families did not qualify for a service even though their children had extensive needs. One professional wondered whether the hospices' fund-raising requirements were to some extent determining their eligibility criteria:

> 'My understanding is that if money is raised publicly for hospices then it is important for them to use phrases like "life-threatened" or "life-limited" – the use of emotive language is important to fund-raising. My concern is that we have families who have very demanding children who can miss out on the sort of care the hospices provide if they stick rigidly to these criteria.'

However, our impression was that hospices are establishing criteria defining the type of children eligible to use the service because of pressure on places rather than concerns about fund-raising.

Hospices need to generate a large proportion of their own funds. At least one of the four hospices faced difficulties with obtaining statutory funding for hospice placements. A lack of agreement between health and social services about funding services could also be problematic.

Although most of the professionals believed that hospices were flexible about age limits and would continue to provide a service to anyone over the age of 19, there was some concern about these young people. Most hospices do currently cater for young adults who have been receiving a service during their childhood. However, some hospice staff indicated that a change of policy could not be ruled out and they were increasingly hesitant about making longer-term or indefinite commitments to families.

Referrals

Three of the four hospices accepted initial requests for help from anyone, though these had to be supported by a formal referral from a medical practitioner. The fourth hospice would take self-referrals without requiring a GP's recommendation. However, records indicated that although 25 per cent of referrals came from a medical practitioner:

- 21 per cent came from social workers;
- 19 per cent from the families themselves;
- 15 per cent from community nurses;
- 9 per cent from education professionals.

Five of the 38 families interviewed had concerns about the referral process, mainly because of fears that they would not be offered a service because of demand for places and, in one case, because the family lived just outside the catchment area.

Variations in who was eligible for a particular hospice's service meant that if families moved to another area where there was a children's hospice, they could not be certain that they would continue to receive a service of this kind. In fact, this *had* happened to one of the families we interviewed.

Other factors which may influence access

Apart from the hospices' own eligibility criteria, access to the service may also be influenced by the ethnic background and socio-economic status of families with disabled children.

Ethnicity

In two of the hospices, the proportion of children from minority ethnic groups was lower than would be expected, given their catchment areas. There were a number of possible reasons for this:

- the service was not publicised sufficiently widely or appropriately within minority ethnic communities so families were unaware of its existence;
- the service was not attractive or appropriate for families from a minority ethnic background;
- families were aware of the service but did not require it.

There was no evidence of translated leaflets about the service at any of the four hospices. However, the presence of staff from minority ethnic groups at one hospice was useful in helping to disseminate information by word of mouth to relevant groups in the community. This service was the only one which had successfully recruited staff from minority ethnic groups and the one which had been most successful in attracting children from them.

All four hospices aimed to serve all sections of the community but two had strong religious foundations which might not be attractive to families from minority ethnic communities – or, indeed, to other families who did not share those religious beliefs.

Whilst the hospices seek to offer a service from a non-denominational stance, even the presence of religious artefacts or symbols may deter some families. Those families who were using hospice care were unlikely to complain about religious artefacts around the buildings since they generally felt extremely grateful for the help they were receiving – help which had often not been offered by others.

Families may be concerned that an all-white staff group would be unwilling or unable to follow their particular cultural and/or religious traditions (Baxter and others, 1990). Indeed, during our interviews with staff, it became clear that hospice workers' cultural awareness varied considerably. Some recognised this as an issue needing to be addressed, but others did not.

One hospice recognised the need to reflect a wider range of cultures through materials, music and decor, even though it was not currently catering for families from minority ethnic backgrounds. This hospice was also working towards conveying more positive images of disability, an issue staff regarded as particularly important for siblings who came to the hospice.

Finally, do families from minority ethnic groups know about hospices but choose not to use them? Given the general public's confusion about the role of hospices (see 'Background' on page 3) and the general absence of multilingual literature and staff, it is probably lack of information rather than rejection of the service per se which leads to the low take-up by families from minority ethnic communities.

Socio-economic status

Research by Gordon, Parker and Loughran (1996) found that poorer families received less support than did other families. Although our research did not focus specifically on the socio-economic status of the families, of the 38 we interviewed, the following information suggested many families were on low incomes and some parents had given up work in order to become full-time carers:

- 29 per cent were single parents;
- only one mother worked (part time) outside the home;
- over 25 per cent of fathers (present) were unemployed;
- 17 per cent of fathers (living with the child) were in manual jobs.

The information we gathered also reinforces previous research findings which have highlighted the difficulty of combining paid employment with caring for a severely disabled child (Baldwin, 1985; Meltzer, Smyth and Robus, 1989; Robinson and Stalker, 1989; Kagan, Lewis and Heaton, 1998).

Older children and young adults

Whilst most hospices were continuing to cater for young adults who had been using their service as children, hospice staff indicated that they were increasingly hesitant about making long-term commitments to families.

Professionals supporting these families were aware that the range of options for short-term care tended to decrease even further as the child reached adulthood. As one of them observed:

> 'Children are surviving longer and there is really no good provision for them . . . [With] this particular family, the child needs more short-term care than they currently get; the service they receive is quite limited, due to the pressure on [the hospice].'

The possibility that support services may become more difficult to access can be an additional burden for families, who are also having to come to terms with the fact that their son's or daughter's condition is unlikely to improve – and may even deteriorate – as they grow up.

The families' use of hospice care

Information on the nature, amount and frequency of use was obtained from two sources:

- analysis of records on 358 children using the hospices between 1 April 1995 and 31 March 1996;
- the interviews with families.

The records search provided the following information about 358 children:

- average number of stays they had per year was 5.3;
- on average children stayed for 40 12-hour sessions a year;
- 78 per cent of their admissions were for planned short-term care;
- 22 per cent were emergency admissions;
- six children had had three or more emergency admissions but given that three of these children had died, the

admissions were probably linked to the child's deteriorating condition;
- children were accompanied by a family member in 14 per cent of admissions.

There was some variation between hospices in:

- the average and maximum number of **stays** they offered;
- the average and maximum number of **12-hour sessions**.

Note. The number of 12-hour sessions was calculated as follows:

day of admission = one session
day of discharge = one session
intervening days = two sessions
arrival one day and discharge the next = three sessions.

One hospice had provided 32 stays to one child and another 20 stays each to three children. However, these individual cases were exceptional and the average number of stays was around five for each of the three hospices catering for larger numbers of children.

Of the 39 children whose families were interviewed:

- the average number of stays per year was seven;
- the average total use per year was 57 12-hour sessions;
- all had had planned short-term care, 95 per cent with a regular pattern of use;
- 30 per cent of children had less than four stays per year;
- **4.5 per cent of children had more than one admission per month.**

There were some variations in the number of hours of care provided. This was because:

- the newest hospice could offer more frequent and longer stays as it was not yet oversubscribed;
- another offered a small number of children more frequent and extensive stays because of their specific circumstances.

On average, children stayed for 40 12-hour sessions a year but in a small number of cases, children had more than 120 days short-term care, exceeding the maximum now allowed under the Children Act (see Chapter 7).

Case study 3: Arun

Arun is ten and lives with his parents and sisters: Lata who is 14 and Savita who is 17. His married sister, Anjana lives nearby. The family live in a small semi-detached house in a large city.

Both Arun's parents were born in India, although his father arrived in the UK as a child and his mother came over 20 years ago when she got married. Arun's dad works full time in the family business nearby, while his mum stays at home. Arun's dad speaks fluent English but his wife only speaks Hindi – the language they use in their home.

Arun has Sandhoff Disease which means he has severe epilepsy, learning difficulties and problems with swallowing. Because an older son died of the same condition eight years ago, Arun's parents are now aware that his condition is progressive. Arun was 'a bright little child' at first and his parents were unaware that he could have inherited the same condition as his brother. They only realised this when he began to display the same symptoms.

The family first heard about the hospice when Arun's older brother was ill, though at this point the family had no idea their eldest son would not get better (especially as the consultant had said they could take him home). Arun's mum was pregnant with Arun and a hospital social worker suggested hospice care which would give the whole family a break. Arun's dad didn't find this easy, particularly since their experience with the hospital had been 'very difficult'.

It took the family a long time to get used to the idea of the hospice but by the time Arun needed it, they already knew the staff and felt more confident at the prospect. Arun has spent a lot of time in hospital and still goes back from time to time. He picks up chest infections quite easily and swallowing has become even more difficult. According to Arun's dad: 'It takes a long time to feed him and he did get very thin at one time'. Tube feeding has been suggested as a future possibility but the family are unsure about it.

Arun is unable to do anything for himself. He needs to be lifted and moved fequently to prevent pressure sores, although last time he was in hospital, his dad remembers, 'he had a bad pressure sore on his back which had become infected'.

Although Arun has no speech, he can let other people know whether he is uncomfortable or hungry by his facial expressions. His dad says Arun is aware of his surroundings and can recognise people he knows.

During the week Arun goes to a special school 12 miles away. According to his dad, Arun 'gets very tired [which is] just unfortunate' because being the first to be collected he is picked up at 7 a.m. and doesn't get home until after 5 p.m.

The hospice has recently employed an Asian outreach worker who vists the family at home and keeps Arun's mum in the picture about her son's stays at the hospice. She has also helped by explaining Arun's condition to his two sisters. Arun's mum and dad particularly appreciate the outreach worker's support.

Arun's older sisters sometimes look after him when they aren't busy with school or college work, but the family receive no help outside the family except a week's hospice care three times a year, so these breaks are very precious to the family. Although his mum still has some concerns about his diet at the hospice, 'Arun seems to enjoy himself and it gives us time to spend with our other children'.

3   Why families use hospices, their expectations and views about hospice care

This chapter focuses on which families use hospices and why, what their expectations are and how they subsequently view the service they receive.

Why families use hospices

There has been relatively little research into why families use hospices (Herd, 1990; Stein and Woolley, 1990). To find some answers to this important question of how families come to use hospices, interviews were conducted with 38 families and with 17 professionals who had referred children to hospices.

There are four broad reasons why families choose, or are directed towards, hospice care:

- positive recommendations;
- unsatisfactory or negative experiences of using other short-term care services;
- inadequate or inappropriate services offered;
- lack of alternatives and barriers to existing provision.

Positive recommendations

Some families had heard positive things about hospice care:

- from other families already using the service;
- through a chance meeting with someone who had indirect contact with a hospice;
- from coverage on regional television programmes or in newspapers;
- from medical consultants and other professionals, including teachers and school nurses.

One family had been contacted by a hospice who had seen them on television.

From the interviews with professionals, it emerged that most considered the service provided by hospices to be superior to that provided elsewhere because they offered one-to-one care, 24-hour cover and support (including accommodation) for the whole family.

Unsatisfactory experiences of other services

One third of the families were using *only* the hospice for short-term care, but others had used a range of other support services including:

- hospitals (4);
- local authority homes/hostels (5);
- family link and fostering schemes (13);
- in-home sitting/care attendants/nursing services (10);
- home helps/family aides (5);
- holiday playschemes (8).

Although some families were no longer using these services, others were continuing to do so alongside hospice care. In certain cases, families had been offered a service but this had been inadequate for their level of need or unsuitable for their particular child.

Despite families' frequently negative experiences of alternatives to hospice care, certain services were mentioned in very positive terms including:

- the home-based nursing assistance one mother was receiving for up to eight hours a day;
- home help and family aides who either took other children to school or who did housework, freeing the parent to care for their disabled child;
- holiday playschemes (though these tended to operate only during the summer).

Hospitals

Only four families had taken up the option of a hospital bed for short-term care. One family no longer sent their child for hospital care and the remaining three said they only used it when desperate. The level of care on hospital wards was generally regarded as poor:

'He is occasionally left "dirty" for long periods in hospital and developed very bad nappy rash as a result.'

'Experience of using hospitals is very different [from the hospice]. Hospitals do not give him anything like as good care as the "normal" children there are given.'

In one case, a child was accommodated on an adult ward, which the family, not surprisingly, considered inappropriate. Hospital staff were seen as unsupportive and parents complained that they were generally expected to stay with the child which meant they had no proper break themselves.

These findings endorse previous research which found that parents were more likely to be dissatisfied with hospital care than with other short-term care facilities (Stalker and Robinson, 1993; ACT and the Royal College of Paediatrics and Child Health, 1997).

Local authority homes/hostels

Five families had used social services' hostels or children's homes for short-term care and four continued to do so, though there were often restrictions on using these facilities (see elsewhere in this section).

Family link and fostering schemes

Thirteen families had used these schemes, nine were still doing so and one had only recently been linked to a family. None were using this service more than once a month. Three families had ceased using this provision, in one case because the support carer was unable to cope with the child's care regime.

One of the professionals interviewed had had poor experiences of placing a child with a family providing short-term fostering:

'Social Services, who do short-term care, set up fostering for this child; unfortunately, each time the child returned from a foster placement she had a chest infection and had to go immediately to hospital as an emergency admission.'

In-home sitting/care attendant and nursing services

Ten families had used these services and one was waiting to start, though only five were still using in-home services at the time of the interviews. In some cases this type of support was problematic because:

- the family home was cramped, making it difficult to accommodate another person, particularly at night;
- the temptation for the substitute carer to ask the family's advice when they were unsure about what needed to be done meant parents could not really relax;
- parents were often very aware of the child's presence if he or she was noisy or had sleeping difficulties which meant they were disturbed.

As one parent commented:

'Family-based short-term care is inadequate for our needs and bringing additional help into the home is not the same.'

Home helps/family aides

Four families were supported in this way but with a fifth family, whose child had been experiencing feeding difficulties, the support had been withdrawn when the feeding improved.

Holiday playschemes

Although all eight families using these indicated they would continue to do so, this service tended to be only available during the summer holidays and occasionally during the spring break.

Offered inadequate or inappropriate services

The majority of families had been offered a **hospital** bed for short-term care but almost unanimously they disliked the idea of their children going into hospital. Many of these young people had already been subjected to a great deal of unpleasant hospital treatment and would therefore associate going into hospital with previous negative experiences. These parental misgivings were echoed by some professionals:

'We are aware that if children like this do go into hospital for a break they often come out more ill, with a hospital-acquired infection, than when they went in – again this makes us reluctant to suggest it as an option. It also puts parents off.'

Several families had been offered short-term care in **social services' homes or hostels** but, as the following comments indicate, had found this provision wanting:

'We recently visited a residential facility for children with disabilities [jointly run by Health and Social Services]; it was very basic and dismal in comparison to the hospice.'

'We did go and see a Social Services short-term care place but it was horrible – we wouldn't let him go there.'

One family had been offered **family-based care** but had refused it because they felt that the support carers were not sufficiently experienced to care for their child, saying:

'The Social Services and Barnardo's short-term care scheme is the only thing available locally; [this is] inadequate for our needs.'

Lack of alternatives and barriers to existing provision

For some families whose children had complex health needs, there appeared to be few options available and for some, referral to the hospice had been in the nature of a 'last resort'. Both parents and professionals mentioned the lack of alternatives which could provide a regular break.

Professionals felt that staff levels in non-hospice services were inadequate and that staff lacked the necessary skills and/or knowledge to carry out certain procedures such as resuscitation or management of complex seizures. As one professional commented:

'There are little or no facilities in the community for these children so the families tend to use the hospices because there is nothing else.'

Although professionals making referrals had many positive things to say about hospices, nevertheless, some questioned the suitability of hospice-based care for children, feeling that a 'specialist unit which is locally based' would be more appropriate.

Parents and professionals identified a number of barriers to using provision other than hospices. Many residential facilities operated **age restrictions** and did not take under-fives. As one professional had discovered:

'The only other [alternative to the hospice] cannot take children under five and there were no foster carers available because of the special needs this child had.'

Families with an **older child** could also encounter problems. One referring professional, for example, decided that family-based care was not appropriate for a particular teenager:

'I don't think it is appropriate to cater for someone of [this child's] age in a family because his needs are such that they wouldn't be able to cope as he gets older [and] these needs increase as he gets larger to handle: it's not so easy for a family to take on an adult.'

The professionals interviewed were aware that the range of options tended to dwindle even further as **children reached adulthood**. As one observed:

'Children are surviving longer and there is no really good provision for them. The cost of equipment to support them in their daily living increases [too] as they grow older.'

The state of the child's health was also an issue. Some parents mentioned that **children had to be 'well'** in order to use social services' facilities and since many of these children have only short periods when they are 'well', access is very restricted.

Some local authorities have adopted **policies on invasive treatments** which prevent carers other than parents, who are not nurses, from undertaking certain treatments. As one professional pointed out:

'Short-term care for children with complex health needs is becoming more of a headache, especially [for] children with gastrostomies. There are problems with the legal side.'

One parent commented on how this excluded them from the option of using family-based care:

'Local social services say they can't place children with invasive therapies with families.'

One of the referring professionals also described the following situation of a child (now using a hospice):

'[the child] is tube-fed, has breathing problems, [and] has severe epilepsy which requires the administration of rectal diazepam. His mother [a lone parent] was not getting any form of short-term care at the time – her family were unable to help. The local social services accommodation would not take children who are tube-fed.

The only option for [the child], given the extensive and complex needs, was a unit staffed by RSCNs [Registered Sick Children's Nurses].'

Parents' expectations

Parents were asked about what they expected from hospice care and Table A5 in the Appendix sets out their detailed responses. The most commonly cited expectations were frequent breaks (47 per cent) and good quality care (29 per cent) – the kind of expectations which any family using short-term care services would be likely to mention (Robinson and Stalker, 1990). Others such as 'good professional care' and 'catering for a wide range of needs' related more specifically to hospice care.

Although 44 per cent of parents said their original expectations of the hospice had been exceeded, 25 per cent said their expectations had not been met which must be a matter of some concern. A common reason for their disappointment was that they were not receiving as much help as they would have liked.

Nearly two thirds of the families had been using the service for more than three years. It was therefore not surprising that many were being offered fewer breaks now as the service had become more well known and overall demand had presumably increased. Nowadays new users are likely to be offered a more limited amount of help from the outset.

Initial impressions

The overwhelming majority of families had been pleasantly surprised by the hospice's facilities, the friendliness of the staff and the generally informal atmosphere. They appreciated the non-clinical atmosphere and non-hierarchical ambience:

'It is not what I expected . . . it's a lot more of a friendly family atmosphere'.

'It's like a hotel with lots of friends . . . there's laughter as well as sadness; everybody is equal. All the families are there with a child who is dying.'

Several people talked about the importance of a non-clinical environment which was often in stark contrast to their previous use of hospitals. Many families had expected the hospice environment to be not unlike that of a hospital. For some the word 'hospice', with its connotations with death and dying (Chadwick, 1993), had also been a source of anxiety.

Being made to feel welcome by the hospice staff was important, helping the families to trust them and feel confident about their child's care. High staffing levels and having a named member of staff available for their child were also important.

Two families had had less positive experiences on their initial visit. In the first instance, the parents still have vivid memories of being actively prepared for their child's death, although they had not requested counselling (and the child is still alive three years later). In the second case, at the time of referral, neither mother nor child spoke or understood any English and the inability of staff to communicate with them was extremely distressing. (Both are now fluent in English and feel confident and competent about communicating with hospice staff.)

Parents' views about hospice care

Parents were asked what they felt were the 'best' and 'worst' aspects of using the hospice and their responses are set out in Tables 3.1 and 3.2.

The opportunity to have a break while their child was receiving good quality care were the two positive aspects most frequently cited, a finding which mirrors those of other studies on short-term care (Robinson and Stalker, 1990; Newitt, Jones and Robinson, 1998). However, for some families, using the hospice also gave them 'peace of mind' and the chance to 'get life into perspective'.

Over a quarter of families had no specific criticisms of the hospice but the 'worst' things cited by some families do have implications for future policy and practice, notably:

- the location of hospices and the distances families had to travel to reach them, indicating that more local provision would be welcome;
- the lack of availability, presumably referring to the frequency with which families were able to use the service.

Overall, then, despite the concerns of a few parents about the quality of care and their guilt about the children being cared for by others, the vast majority of parents were extremely positive about the service provided.

Table 3.1   Best things about using a hospice

The 'best things'	Number of respondents mentioning*	%
The break	16	42.1
The excellent/safe care	8	21.1
Time for other children	6	15.8
Knowing that 'X' is happy	5	13.2
Peace of mind	4	10.5
Good facilities/nice place for 'X'	4	10.5
Time for self	4	10.5
Knowing it is there in case of emergency	3	7.9
Knowing you're not alone – support of other families	3	7.9
Interesting outings/holidays	2	5.3
Staff are friends	1	2.6
Provided what I needed	1	2.6
Been able to get life into perspective	1	2.6
Can go on public transport	1	2.6
Pretend we're normal for a few days	1	2.6

*Not cumulative, parents could cite more than one response

Table 3.2   Worst things about using a hospice

The 'worst things'	Number of respondents mentioning*	%
The travel, owing to distance	10	26.3
Lack of availability	4	10.5
'Letting go'	3	7.9
Having to book so far ahead	2	5.3
Worry that care is not good enough	2	5.3
The guilt (which continues)	2	5.3
Coming to terms with need for hospice	2	5.3
Seeing other children deteriorate (realising own child will too)	2	5.3
Lack of education/stimulation	2	5.3
Loss of 'X's' routine	1	2.6
Accepting the need for help	1	2.6
Grandparent disapproved	1	2.6
Child transferred to hospice to die and did not	1	2.6
None	10	26.3

*Not cumulative, parents could cite more than one response

Case study 4: Clara

Clara is 18-years-old. An only child, she lives with her mum and dad, both of whom have retired. The family lives in an inner city area, in a small terraced house where Clara's dad was born.

Clara has Down's syndrome and epilepsy. She also has a progressive heart condition and is waiting for a heart-lung transplant, though her dad is pessimistic about whether she will ever get one. Clara is physically quite frail; she tires easily and uses oxygen to help her breathe. Her condition has deteriorated over the last two or three years before which she was, in her mum's words: 'a bubbly and chirpy character, always up to mischief'.

During the week, Clara attends the local special school just around the corner, though because she spent a lot of time in hospital when younger, she didn't start school until she was seven-years-old.

Clara communicates by using a mixture of speech and Makaton (a sign language) and the family have been involved with a group at school which supports parents whose children use signing.

Clara really enjoys school and has lots of friends there. She is particularly interested in computing, has her own computer at home and would eventually like to work as a secretary. She also belongs to her local Gateway club, and she has been on their holidays, except for the last two years when she hasn't been well enough. Horse-riding is one of her passions and something she still insists on doing even when, according to her mum, 'she's not feeling too special'. She is also keen on acting and has been in the school show every year since she was 11.

Eight years ago, Clara's mum was diagnosed with breast cancer and the question arose of where Clara would live while her mum was in hospital having treatment as her dad was working full time as a long-distance lorry driver. There didn't seem to be anywhere suitable until a friend of Clara's mum mentioned the children's hospice.

The family asked their GP if there might be a place at the hospice for Clara and she has been staying there for short breaks ever since, though demand for places means the number of breaks has been reduced over the last two years.

Clara generally enjoys her hospice stays, although she gets bored if there aren't any other teenagers staying or other children are 'really ill'. The begining and end of the breaks can be difficult sometimes. If either of her parents are ill, Clara worries and tends to 'kick up a fuss' if she is due to go to the hospice. And according to her mum, she 'gets spoiled' there and it takes her a while to settle back home again.

As Clara gets older, her parents worry about the future, especially since Clara will be leaving school next year. They are both less physically-able to look after her and feel that without the hospice breaks they would be lost. Her mum also realises that the hospice is 'tightening up on who they take' and though Clara can still go there at the moment they have no idea about what may happen in future.

4 The children's experiences

Introduction

This chapter aims to provide a picture of the children's experiences of staying in a hospice: how they coped with leaving and being reunited with their families; how they spent their time during their stays; and how they interacted with staff as well as with the other children.

We built up this picture through spending time in the hospices. The interviews with parents also helped us develop a fuller picture and the records search provided data on the activities available to the children.

Although the children themselves were not formally interviewed, at each of the hospices some of the children struck up conversations with the observers. They chatted to us while involved in an activity and the more outgoing ones came and sat beside us or asked us to participate in a game or task.

The remainder of this chapter focuses on how the children:

- coped with stays away from home;
- interacted with staff;
- spent their time.

The children's experiences of going away

Previous research has highlighted the incidence of home-sickness amongst children using short-term care services (Oswin, 1984; Robinson, 1986; Robinson and Stalker, 1990).

When asked how they felt their child reacted to the separation, the majority of parents said that when they saw their child at the hospice he or she had appeared to be enjoying it ('she doesn't want to come home'). A few were unsure, some parents commenting that they felt their child was 'simply not aware of their environment'. However, a small number of children were said to be unhappy. Parents made the following comments:

> '[She] is much noisier when she is at the hospice . . . she cries more and is glad to be picked up and taken home.'

> '[He is not happy] because he is too active and too bright [and on one occasion he had been] asking for his mum for ages.'

One child was said to be unhappy sometimes if the stay was for longer than one or two nights, so the parents had stopped using the service for longer stays.

Another child did not eat properly while at the hospice. Although the parents did not think this meant he was unhappy, the food at the hospice was of a good quality and, as they commented, their son ate well at home:

> 'Basically [he] only eats properly at home . . . he always seems quite happy – he loves the trips out and the activities – but he is always ready to come home – maybe because he is hungry.'

On the other hand, some parents felt the hospice stays had been very beneficial for their child who had made progress while there:

> 'We have occasional sleep problems, but on the whole he is better, more alert, when he's been there; he seems to have made some progress each time he comes home; it is [the hospice] that have done that for him.'

From interviews with the parents it was, not surprisingly, the outgoing, confident and more sociable children who enjoyed their stays, whereas the timid or physically vulnerable children coped less well and could find stays away from home stressful.

The observers' informal conversations tended to be with the more outgoing children and, not surprisingly, most appeared to feel at home and were very positive about their experiences at the hospice.

When it came to leaving their child at the hospice, only two families said their child seemed reluctant to be left. One said their child sometimes got upset and the other commented:

> 'He's difficult because he doesn't want to leave the family – he becomes obstinate.'

For the children, returning home after time spent away from the family seemed more difficult. Nearly half the families mentioned difficulties including:

- the onset of physical problems such as constipation or digestive upsets;
- disturbed sleep patterns;
- more demanding, clingy or awkward behaviour.

Comments about their child's reactions included:

'For two to three weeks on returning home he behaves very spoilt.'

'He is distressed on returning home; he is very disorientated and confused. I feel [the hospice] could have prepared him better; they are not always honest with him.'

Another parent noted that she was 'sent to Coventry' by her daughter for a while after the hospice visits.

A final, but important aspect of how children coped, was raised by two parents who commented that staying in the hospice had been more difficult for the child than staying in family settings:

'She does not react this way [being demanding] after staying at [family-based carer's home].'

'He has no problems when he stays at Grandma's.'

Staff–children interactions

The way staff and volunteers interacted with the children was obviously important in terms of how the children experienced their stays at the hospice. Although staff talked to the children, only a minority of the children could respond verbally, and mostly only in a rather limited fashion.

The 39 children whose parents were interviewed communicated as follows:

- facial expressions (12);
- sounds (7);
- mood (for example happy or sad) (6);
- speech, odd words (though meaning not always appropriate), and in two cases combined with signing (6);
- cries if unhappy (but won't necessarily smile if happy) (5);

- eye movements (2);
- Makaton/BSL (1).

Communication is not only an issue in relation to staff; it does, of course, have wider implications, particularly in trying to understand how the children reacted to staying in the hospice.

In all the hospices, staff usually talked to the children to encourage them to undertake various activities, although in some instances they also had to physically assist the child or demonstrate the activity in question.

Children were generally encouraged to make choices and be involved in whatever they wished, within normal standards of behaviour. If they wanted to do something that was not possible, staff carefully explained the reasons.

However, there were instances where staff appeared not to know how to communicate with a particular child, particularly if that child was a relatively new user of the service. This was endorsed by a small number of parents:

> 'I don't feel the hospice staff always make enough effort to communicate with her.'

> 'We understand him best . . . we haven't seen any staff using Makaton [which was the child's main method of communication].'

At the same time, parents recognised that it takes time for staff to learn to communicate effectively with an individual child:

> 'He has been going [to the hospice] for a long time so they are aware of his needs, but this may not be the case with someone new.'

One of the issues we were particularly concerned about was the continuity of care which the children received from staff during their hospice stays, particularly as they often had complex needs, requiring extensive intimate care. We were also aware of the importance families generally attach to having a nominated keyworker, even though they are often not assigned one (While, Citrone and Cornish, 1996).

We therefore asked parents whether their child had a keyworker or link-worker at the hospice and if that person spent much time with them. We found that:

- 64 per cent of the children had a keyworker or link-worker;
- 18 per cent did not;
- 18 per cent of families didn't know.

Of the 64 per cent whose child did have a keyworker or link-worker:

- nearly half thought their child did not spend much time with this person; and,
- just over a quarter did not know who the keyworker was.

The following comment from one parent was typical in demonstrating that the system was not as effective as it might be:

> 'Yes [there is a keyworker system], but the keyworker keeps changing . . . often, they are not even on duty or the keyworker is the person in charge so they cannot spend much individual time with the children.'

This quotation highlights the difficulties managers experience in operating an effective keyworker system. Parents recognised the desirability of having a known person to provide the extensive intimate care these children usually needed but only a minority knew whether their child had any choice about who attended to their needs and whether preferences for a male or female carer were met.

However, we were pleased to find that in most situations children's care needs were dealt with in a sensitive and discreet manner. Personal needs were attended to in privacy, usually by the carer allocated to that particular child that day or that shift. If a staff member was less than discreet this was quickly pointed out by another member of staff and the situation rectified.

How the children spent their time

Table 4.1 lists the range of activities which the hospices offered in 1995–6 and the take-up on these. The range is broad. Some were specifically 'therapeutic' such as physiotherapy, sessions on signing and other communication techniques and use of a multi-sensory room. Others were more purely recreational such as day trips and outings. Others could be described as 'educational' but also incorporated elements of 'play' such as video and computer games, arts and crafts, and play activities.

The table shows an impressive range of activities, but take-up for some was very low. This was reflected in the observers' findings. There were few examples of planned activities at any

Table 4.1   Range of therapeutic activities on offer and 'take-up'

Type of therapeutic activity	Number of children engaged in the activity (n=358)*	%
Physiotherapy	154	44.1
Play activities	139	39.8
Hydrotherapy including Jacuzzi	123	35.2
Educational activities	63	18.1
Multi-sensory room/snoezelen	63	18.1
Music	48	13.8
Massage	39	11.2
Videos and computer games	38	10.9
Aromatherapy	19	5.4
Day trips/outings	10	2.9
Arts and crafts	7	2.0
Multi-gym	4	1.2
Signing/communication techniques	1	0.3
Make-up	1	0.3
Cooking	1	0.3
Missing information	7	2.0

*Not cumulative as children could participate in several activities

of the hospices, although there were some one-to-one activities with children when a full complement of staff was on duty.

Examples of group activities observed included:

- a structured music session involving all the children (except those who clearly chose to opt out), where the most severely disabled children were encouraged and, where necessary, helped to participate by staff;
- a trip to the local swimming pool which most children went on and where all the children were encouraged to swim or float with as much assistance as they required;
- an outing for the more 'able' children, the more dependent children remaining at the hospice.

The first two examples demonstrate how it *is* possible to organise inclusive activities for severely disabled children.

All the hospices had an outside play or recreational area and at one hospice the children were actively encouraged to run around or ride bicycles. At one hospice, the children who needed the exercise and the few boisterous children who needed to burn off excess energy, were encouraged to play outside so they would not harm the more physically frail children.

Children not participating in organised activities, spent their time in unstructured play. This was often on their own, apart from occasional interaction with staff, though many needed prompting and directing in order to occupy themselves.

How the children occupied their time depended to some extent on their age (as well as how 'able' they were). Play options for babies and younger children were limited, and younger children tended to remain in one area or room for long periods unless there was sufficient staffing for them to have individual attention.

The older children, like many teenagers, tended to occupy themselves with things like video and computer games rather than more 'soothing' therapies. The older and more mobile children tended to come and go very much as they pleased. The informal conversations with some of the older children revealed that they were a bit bored at times, particularly if the rest of the group were considerably younger or significantly more disabled than they were. The lack of a peer group seemed important to some of these older children who tended to deal with this by opting out – retreating to their bedrooms to listen to music, for example. As in other settings, where a peer group is not available, teenagers tended to interact with younger members of staff as a 'substitute'.

During 'free play' periods, children unable to occupy themselves usually sat in their wheelchairs or lay on mats – usually with a video or TV programme playing in the room.

The level of activity tended to be influenced by the number of staff on duty and on what was happening during a particular shift, although, not surprisingly, it was the least able children who were most affected by staff shortages. As staff at one hospice commented, it was these children, particularly if they were very quiet and passive, who tended to miss out. When there were sufficient staff on duty, children of all ages and degrees of impairment received more attention and stimulus from staff:

'The need for one-to-one care for most of the children was demonstrated by the amount of time spent by one carer with a severely disabled child in the multi-sensory room. Sensory stimulation was available through touching and assisting the child to touch "tactile response" objects in the room.'

The more severely disabled children also presented the greatest challenge to staff in terms of finding appropriate stimulation – a challenge not confined to hospices. A few parents also expressed concern at the level of stimulation provided:

'I am concerned that she doesn't always get enough stimulation at the hospice.'

'He needs more stimulation and play; the staff are often sitting around and the children are left to their own devices.'

Where children were staying at the hospice during term-time, school would obviously occupy a large part of the day. However, although nearly half the school-age children did attend school during their hospice stays, the remainder did not. This was generally because the hospice was too far from their school. Three children were not receiving any formal education: one family felt the child was too frail to attend school, one child had not started school because of ill-health and in the third case the LEA was having difficulty finding a place which could cater for the child's high level of need.

Mealtimes

Mealtimes are important in any context – whether in the family or elsewhere – and the observers participated in at least one meal each time they were at a hospice. A number of aspects were considered:

- how mealtimes were organised;
- which children participated;
- how children and staff interacted;
- what foods were on offer.

Not all the hospices had organised mealtimes where everyone sat at table together regardless of whether they ate ordinary food or were tube-fed. In three of the four hospices, there was at least one tube-fed child who the staff considered did not need to be present during mealtimes when the other children were eating.

In one hospice there were no mealtimes as such: each child had a personal feeding regimen so the children rarely ate at the same time; and in another, most children who were tube-fed or required liquidised food, were fed in a room adjacent to the one where staff and the remaining children were eating. In another hospice, the mealtime *was* a social opportunity for everyone and tube-fed children were generally included at table along with the other staff, visitors and the other children.

The decision to exclude some children is questionable since many of the children could undoubtedly have been given tasters of food, even if they could not swallow, and would thus have been included (Carroll and Reilly, 1996; Townsley and Robinson, 1997b).

On the whole, mealtimes were reasonably pleasant with staff and children interacting well, though in one hospice staff sometimes popped in and out rather than sitting at table with the children. Observers noted one or two less happy occasions. On one occasion a child became frustrated, perhaps because of her communication difficulties, and began throwing food but this was handled well and the situation did not escalate. Frequently all or most of the children required help with eating.

The quality of food on offer between the hospices was variable. In one, there was a heavy reliance on convenience goods which, though probably appealing to the children, was not particularly nutritious.

Sometimes staff were under pressure to produce a meal quickly because kitchen staff were absent and in these instances too, the food was less nutritious and interesting than usual.

Two of the hospices catered for special dietary needs, providing vegetarian, halal and kosher meals, always providing an alternative when they were needed. Other special diets were provided if necessary in all the hospices.

The mix of children

Few of the hospices seemed to routinely plan non-emergency admissions on the basis of achieving the best possible 'mix' of children in terms of their ages and degree of frailty. However, where this happened, the grouping could be compromised by an emergency admission of a child of a different age or with a different level of need.

There were often different age groups. At one hospice, for example, the age range of children at one time was six months to 14 years and the children were clearly incompatible in terms of their age and behaviour. In all the hospices, physically frail children were sometimes in residence alongside more boisterous children.

This mix of children meant that young and/or frail children were in danger of being walked on or hit by other children whose behaviour was challenging, particularly when staffing levels were low or staff were preoccupied with an ill child or a death. As one observer noted:

> Staff were very stretched and the mix of children was very demanding. There was a small baby who didn't need much doing for him but who couldn't be left alone because of vulnerability from other children. One girl was particularly difficult and kept hitting other children. All the children's needs could clearly not be met by the available staff.

One parent also mentioned a couple of occasions where a very active child had sat on her child who is blind and physically immobile – a clearly frightening experience for him.

When staff were physically and emotionally stretched there was less careful monitoring of the frail children who really needed one-to-one supervision. Staff tended to be reactive, rather than proactive, at these times, with vulnerable children having to be 'rescued' from larger and more boisterous children.

Although some parents said they trusted the hospices to care for their frail children because someone was with them 'all the time', clearly this was not always the case. Sometimes when this happened and the family was also staying at the hospice, then they would become involved in keeping an eye on both their own and other people's children.

Case study 5: Pete

Pete, who is six, lives with his parents, three-year-old sister, Lily and eight-year-old brother Jack. The family lives on a large new housing estate on the edge of a town. Pete's mum used to work as a community nurse, but after Pete's birth had to give that up to look after him. His dad is currently unable to work as he is awaiting surgery to correct a recently diagnosed heart condition.

Pete's parents have never been given a diagnosis for their son, but they knew when he was born that he had a lot of problems and was not expected to survive. Pete is severely disabled. He has a cleft palate, severe learning difficulties, heart problems and epilepsy. At times he has what his mum and dad describe as 'breath holding attacks' (which are linked to his medical condition). Because of his impairments, he has to be tube-fed.

According to his mum, Pete is usually quite contented, but when he's frustrated he hits or bites himself, which his parents find very upsetting. He has a limited number of facial expressions, indicating whether he is happy or sad and if annoyed will turn his head away.

Pete attends a local special school, though he has a lot of time off for sickness. He is very susceptible to infections, and more than once has come home from being in hospital for a few days for tests – ending up, as his mum says, 'more ill than before'. This is one of the main reasons why his parents are reluctant to let him stay anywhere where he might pick up an infection.

For a couple of years, Pete did use a short-term care unit run by social services but that was stopped because of the complexity of his needs, especially the tube feeding and administration of rectal diazepam after a bad fit. Pete's mum and dad felt quite angry that *they* were being expected to provide a high level of care, while at the same time social services were not able to do so.

A couple of times a month, Pete's parents can go out for the evening when a voluntary organisation provides a sitter but it was their GP who suggested that the hospice could give the family a longer break.

About a year ago, Pete started going to the hospice for a few days every six to eight weeks. His mum is impressed with the facilities and feels she has a good rapport with the staff.

The only drawback about using the hospice is the distance. Pete's dad has been unable to drive since his heart condition was diagnosed, and since the hospice is 40 miles away, getting there and back is now a major exercise. Pete's mum doesn't drive so a neighbour drives the family's car.

Journeys are not easy anyway. Pete finds the journey upsetting: he finds it difficult to sit comfortably in the car and suffers from travel sickness. The family also have to transport things like Pete's 'special chair' and his buggy and other bits and pieces which make his stays at the hospice more comfortable.

In spite of these complications, Pete seems to enjoy being at the hospice and responds well to having more people around him. He likes the multi-sensory room and the hospice staff continue with the aromatherapy oils his mum uses at home.

When enough staff are around, Pete can go into the hydrotherapy pool though he doesn't like it if there are too many people and his face gets splashed. Pete also enjoys being outdoors – especially in windy weather – and the hospice staff take the children out a lot when it's fine.

For his first stay, all Pete's family stayed too but now he usually stays on his own. This gives Pete more one-to-one attention and gives his parents and Jack and Lily 'the chance to do things as a family without having to plan down to the smallest detail where we go and whether the place will be accessible for Pete'. Both parents are confident that their son is well cared for at the hospice and that they will be contacted if there are any concerns.

5 The families' experiences at the hospices

Introduction

Hospices offer a service not only to children but to their families as well. In this chapter, we focus on:

- whether or not families stayed at the hospice;
- families' experiences at the hospices (including support offered to parents who did not stay);
- the siblings' experiences;
- families and hospice staff.

Families' choice of whether to stay

The range of facilities and services offered to families varied between the hospices. The hospices had differing approaches to accommodating families. One hospice could accommodate families but staff tried to persuade parents to take a rest from their caring role and accommodation was very basic for those who do choose to stay.

At the other end of the spectrum, another hospice had purpose-built and well equipped accommodation which could cater for more than one family at a time and children's friends could also stay. The provision was separate from the children's accommodation, allowing families to control their level of involvement with the hospice. In addition, staff would look after siblings if the parents wished.

From hospice records, it appeared that one or more family members accompanied the children on 14 per cent of their stays and more detailed information from the interviews with 38 families revealed that:

- 10 per cent of mothers 'usually' or 'always' accompanied their child;

- 10 per cent of mothers 'sometimes' stayed;
- 8 per cent of mothers rarely stayed;
- 85 per cent of fathers and 72 per cent of mothers never stayed with their child.

Families had often stayed when their child had first used the hospice, and it was a minority who stayed regularly after that.

Just over half the parents interviewed said that staying at the hospice would prevent them having a complete break. There were other reasons why families did not stay:

- the hospice was too far from the family home which would cause problems with work and school commitments;
- the break enabled them to spend more time with other family members;
- the child did not want family members to stay;
- the family said 'we don't want to'.

Families' experiences at the hospices

Welcoming visitors is an important part of the hospice philosophy. We saw some families receiving a very warm and positive welcome from staff, who greeted them, offered tea or coffee, found them a seat and gave them the opportunity to talk if they wished to do so. These visiting families were well attended to and helped to feel at ease.

However, this was not always the case. Parents could sometimes seem rather neglected, even when plenty of staff were on duty. In one instance, when two parents arrived looking rather uneasy, the television was playing loudly and only one of the care staff interacted with the parents. Observers also noted on one occasion that:

> No one seemed to try and put the mother at ease so she sat and watched television

and on another that:

> [The] staff member removed [the] child from [the] mother and the child was distressed by this.

Despite these variations (which did not always depend on staffing levels), helpful and supportive interactions between staff and families *were* seen in all four hospices, as the following observations demonstrate:

The bereaved family left mid-morning. This was an emotional time for everyone but it was handled with the utmost sensitivity.

The staff were welcoming and spent time explaining about the child's condition.

Parents seemed involved and at home.

Where parents were staying at the hospice, they were often very involved in hospice life, with staff not only caring for the children but supporting the families as well:

There was a real sense of sharing, with parents being supported and also offering support themselves by caring for their families' children.

Hospices usually offered families a range of facilities and during the interviews families mentioned the following (though they had not necessarily used them):

- counselling (14);
- support groups (7);
- general facilities (3);
- aromatherapy (2);
- use of hydrotherapy pool (2);
- social groups (2).

Hospices generally offer support to families, either through counselling or parents' groups, and this is usually regardless of whether or not families choose to stay at the hospice. Although the extent to which families used counselling was not clear, just over two thirds of the families had some form of contact with other parents using the same hospice including:

- informal social contact (44 per cent);
- hospice-run parents' group (10 per cent);
- hospice-run social events (5 per cent).

Other contact with the hospice included informal contact during stays and telephone conversations to discuss bookings.

The relatively small numbers of families attending hospice support groups may well be because of the travel involved when parents were not staying there, rather than for other reasons. However, it is also possible that parents view the hospice as providing a break from being a parent/carer. These parents, who are providing round-the-clock care for their disabled child may also be simply too exhausted to attend such groups.

Families who stayed at the hospice were asked how much they were involved in their child's care and whether this suited them. Thirty families had stayed at least once, most were involved to some extent in their child's care and the majority said this was what they wanted, though two said they had been more involved than they had wanted to be. Only two families said they had no involvement (in one case because of their other children's needs).

The siblings' experiences

In seven families, a sibling had continued to accompany their disabled brother or sister after the first stay.

Other studies (Hochstadt and Yost, 1991; Powell and Gallagher, 1993; While, Citrone and Cornish, 1996) have looked at the impact on children of having a disabled or ill sibling and their findings are echoed in the comment made by one parent in this study who '[felt] quite strongly that brothers and sister should not stay'. A period of time apart from their disabled siblings could allow the non-disabled child or young person to spend time with their own friends and have some individual attention from parents without the added responsibility of caring for a disabled child.

However, some non-disabled siblings did stay. In over half the cases, the sibling had chosen to stay; in other instances parents had suggested the idea; and with two families the hospice had suggested that the sibling's presence would be helpful.

Finally, two families had children with the same condition and both children would stay at the hospice together, giving the parents a much needed break.

Hospice staff and families

Previous studies have highlighted the lack of information about services and about their own child when he or she is using a service (Quine and Pahl, 1989; Robinson and Stalker, 1990; Green and Murton, 1993). Of the parents we interviewed:

- 64 per cent said they had adequate information about developments in the hospice;
- 82 per cent said they had enough information about their child's stays.

However, less than two thirds of parents had met with hospice staff to discuss their child's care and in over two thirds of these meetings no external professional was present to advocate for the child's needs, plan future care and generally broaden the agenda beyond that of hospice care. Given some of the children's reactions to their hospice stays (see Chapter 4), meetings to discuss these – perhaps in the form of regular review meetings – would have been useful.

Despite the infrequency of formal meetings, most families felt they could talk to staff about anything to do with their child's care, however minor it might seem:

- 87 per cent of families always 'felt comfortable';
- the remainder 'usually' or 'sometimes' felt comfortable;
- one family 'rarely' felt comfortable talking to staff.

Although each hospice had a formal complaints procedure, less than a quarter of parents knew about it. However, in the event of a complaint:

- 66 per cent of parents would raise the issue with the manager;
- 10 per cent would talk to a member of staff;
- 10 per cent would talk to their child's keyworker;
- 14 per cent did not know who they would approach.

Parents generally regarded hospice staff in a very positive light. For these parents, the best thing about the hospice was:

'Knowing that [my child] is being cared for as well or better than at home. They are experienced and know what they're doing.'

and

'The main difference [between the hospice and other services] is that I have the confidence to totally hand my child over.'

Although only a proportion of hospice staff were qualified nurses, parents tended to view all the staff as trained professionals whom they could trust:

'They are all qualified nurses, most having worked with children.'

Case study 6: Charlotte

Charlotte, who is 20, lives with her mother in a semi-detached house in the large village where her mum grew up. Her parents separated when she was five-years-old because her father 'couldn't cope with the situation' and, although he only lives 30 miles away, he has no contact with his daughter. Charlotte's mum used to work part time but had to give up her job when Charlotte left school last year.

Charlotte has severe cerebral palsy and is unable to move without help. She needs to be fed, and has an indwelling catheter which leaves her prone to urinary infections. She also has epilepsy though this is mostly well controlled unless she is otherwise unwell.

Charlotte started going to the hospice about 12 years ago and currently spends three or four days there every couple of months.

Charlotte doesn't speak, though she seems to understand what is being said, and when happy or excited will squeal loudly. However, she is also very shy and can get very embarrassed when her personal care needs are being attended to. According to her mum, Charlotte 'definitely prefers women to men when it comes to having a bath or going to the toilet' and, unless there's an emergency her mum always makes sure that staff know Charlotte is to be cared for by female staff which, now that she is no longer a child, is more appropriate.

Charlotte enjoys listening to music – 'the louder the better' according to her mum. She also enjoys being in the water 'because she can move her arms and legs around and float . . . and would probably stay in [the water] all day if you let her'. Hospice staff take the children to the local pool if there are enough of them on duty, which helps compensate for the fact that Charlotte can no longer use the pool at her old school.

As Charlotte leaves her teenage years behind, the hospice has become her and her mother's main support. Since leaving school, Charlotte has spent most of her time at home. According to her mum, social services have not managed to come up with anything that would meet her needs during the day.

Charlotte's mother occasionally goes out shopping or meets friends whilst Charlotte's grandmother comes over. The pair of them enjoy their time together, and Charlotte particularly likes being in the kitchen while her grandma cooks and chats. However, her grandmother can no longer lift her and doesn't feel confident enough to use the hoist, so Charlotte's mum can only be out for fairly brief periods.

Charlotte is now 'quite a handful to lift', according to her mum, and this, together with her generally increasing care needs, means she no longer spends one weekend a month with another family. Owing to Charlotte's weight and her mum's resulting back problems, the family has been supplied with a hoist but it takes up most of the living room and is not portable, making it impossible for Charlotte to have regular stays with another family.

Not surprisingly, both Charlotte and her mum appreciate the hospice's support. At 20, though, Charlotte is now over the hospice's official upper age limit. Her social worker is investigating possible short-term care in a social services unit in the nearby town. However, her mum is uncertain about this alternative option because 'they have less staff than the hospice and they aren't trained nurses'.

6 The staff and volunteers

This chapter is about the staff and volunteers who worked in the four hospices. While mainly based on interviews with 12 staff, it also draws on the interviews with families and referring professionals, and the observation periods.

Of the 12 members of staff interviewed:

- one was a senior manager with no direct involvement in care;
- most of the others were caring directly for the children;
- four were responsible for volunter recruitment and support or staff training and education.

Some managers saw their job as encompassing a number of different roles including managing other staff, educator and, when necessary, using counselling skills. However, in those hospices which had been open longer, functions such as staff training or counselling tended to have been hived off into separate posts. Although none of the staff interviewed made any critical comments about their workload, managers in the newer hospices implied that they found these multiple roles demanding.

Staff views on the role of the hospice

Asked what they saw as the hospice's main purpose and how they felt it benefited the children who used it, staff responses were fairly consistent. Although not everyone was equally clear about the eligibility criteria, they viewed the hospice as a place giving 'support through respite' to families whose children have life-limiting or terminal conditions. Other benefits mentioned included:

- providing disabled children with a new environment;

- 'spoiling' the children and enabling them to do things which were not possible at home;
- enabling non-disabled siblings to spend more time with their parents.

One manager highlighted the informal aspects of hospice care which she felt were unlikely to be found in other settings where severely disabled children were likely to spend their time:

> 'In hospital they wear uniforms whereas here we don't. In the hospice the care can be arranged exactly as the parents wish. They can have everything they want for their child. We are able to provide the same sort of care that could be provided at home.'

Organisation of staffing

The care team

Hospices are autonomous bodies and, when recruiting staff, can decide for themselves what qualifications and skills they are looking for. The extent to which they recruited qualified nurses varied. The ratio of nursing to non-nursing staff during a day shift could be anything from 1:4 to 1:1, although staff interviewed said that more staff could be brought in to work if the particular needs of the children in residence made that necessary.

At night all the hospices generally had two staff on duty, one of whom would be a qualified nurse. This arrangement varied, though, with extra staff being brought in if there was a seriously ill or dying child staying at the hospice.

Bank (or casual) staff

Nurses and care workers, usually people who were employed elsewhere, were sometimes brought in to work on a casual basis as bank staff. These arrangements seemed far from ideal as it was not always possible to find suitably experienced staff at short notice, despite the fact that some hospices had extensive lists of casual staff.

Staffing levels

During the observation periods we recorded the staffing and volunteer levels and ratio of staff/volunteers to children. The numbers of staff, volunteers, disabled children and siblings are given in Table 6.1.

At times staff were under a great deal of pressure, particularly if a significant proportion of the children required a great deal of attention or more vulnerable children had to be protected from other rather boisterous or challenging young people (see Chapter 4, 'The mix of children').

The extent to which staff were able to give individual children – and their parents – undivided attention depended on two factors: the ratio of staff to children; and the extent of the children's needs.

More rarely, there were also occasions when the staff: child ratios were unnecessarily high: when prearranged admissions were cancelled because of children's illness.

Table 6.1   Numbers of staff, volunteers, disabled children and siblings

	Staff	Volunteers	Disabled children	Siblings
Aster House				
Day 1	5	0	4	0
Day 2	5	0	2	0
Day 3	3	0	2	0
Begonia House				
Day 1	8	1	7	1
Day 2	6	0	8	1
Day 3	6	2	6	0
Cherry Blossoms				
Day 1	5	0	6	5
Day 2	4	4	5	5
Day 3	5	2	5	4
Daisy Way				
Day 1	5	0	6	1
Day 2	5	1	6	1
Day 3	3	0	7	1

Shift systems

The length of time staff were on duty varied, but while short shifts might have disrupted the continuity of the children's care, some people were working very long shifts:

Some staff towards the end of a twelve-and-a-half hour shift appeared tired (not surprisingly) and energy levels [were] lower. Staff said they were ready to finish by then.

Where the hospice's policy was that staff and children ate together, that meant staff had no lunch break and no designated rest periods either. This is contrary to the spirit of the EEC Working Time Directive which came into force in October 1998 so it is likely that practices in this respect will have to change.

Teamwork

The hospices generally adopted a teamwork approach, although maintaining this could be difficult if staff were severely overstretched.

In practice, teamwork arrangements were more or less formal. In one hospice, for example, the staff group was divided into two teams, each catering for a small group of children. Staff communicated with each other regularly throughout the shift and assisted each other with activities.

In another hospice the arrangements were not as formalised but there was a general sharing of responsibilities and sense of teamwork. As the observer noted:

Everyone seemed to know what needed doing without much open discussion about who does what.

However, this harmonious working appears to have been jeopardised when staffing levels were low. As one of the researchers noted during observations:

Insufficient staff today to allow teamwork. [My]self and other observer ended up in sole charge of individual children at one time.

In one hospice, the observers noted that the nurse in charge did not appear to know that the nursing director was away for a few days which raises questions about the effectiveness of internal communications, if not working practices.

At certain points, tension between staff was observed, sometimes where there was a handover period between two shifts. At one hospice, for example, the observer noted that 'the night nurse was rather hostile to[wards] a younger day staff nurse at handover.' At other times, staff hinted at tensions within the staff group either because professional groups held differing values or because of differences of opinion about how to care for the children. However, tensions of these kinds were not observed directly.

Regarding three hospices, the observers commented positively about their teamwork (even though this could be difficult to maintain if staff were overstretched). In the fourth case, there were too few children to assess this aspect of the service.

Staff support and development

Support

Children's hospices are generally relatively small, isolated units. Supporting children and their families who are often experiencing considerable stress and intermittent crises in their lives, is stressful for staff too.

Aside from the families' 'agendas', there are stresses inherent in children's hospice work: not only are staff having to face bereavements but the added strains of working with profoundly disabled children and the challenges of supporting those with little or no recognised form of communication.

If staff themselves do not ensure they have sufficient opportunities to relax away from the job, they are in danger of becoming tense or anxious. Alternatively, they may deal with the stress involved by 'cutting off' and becoming unmotivated.

Staff recognised the need for support from colleagues if they, in turn, were to provide a good service to the families:

'The pressure can build up and then people need to be able to offload [on] to colleagues.'

Two managers emphasised the importance of external support. Some staff had access to an independent counselling service, for example. However, staff did not always find it easy to avail themselves of this kind of help:

'The hardest part is getting people to acknowledge that they are finding things difficult and use [the counselling service]. Because of the work we do we like to think it's okay, [and that] we can cope, even when we can't.'

Some referring professionals echoed these comments, expressing genuine concerns about the ability of some hospice staff to cope with the continually stressful nature of the work.

The Association of Children's Hospices offered some support to senior staff with quarterly meetings to discuss issues of shared concern. However, when the research was being undertaken only two of the four hospices belonged to ACH. (Three are now members.) Managers in the other two had arranged regular contact with local hospital staff or had made informal contact with other children's hospices.

Training opportunities

In all the hospices, staff had regular training opportunities, and in contrast to many other services, three managers said their training budget was adequate. Two hospices closed the service to allow training to take place. Events included:

- training on specific topics or programmes of care, using external trainers;
- NVQ programmes with trained staff acting as assessors;
- opportunities to attend external courses;
- support to undertake relevant degree courses.

The following gaps in training were also identified by hospice staff:

- cultural awareness;
- disability awareness;
- working with severely impaired children;
- communication methods;
- ethical issues;
- grief and loss;
- adolescence;
- HIV/AIDS;
- training focused on an individual child's needs.

Some hospices had reciprocal training arrangements with other hospices or hospital units; in one hospice, staff were able to undertake hospital visits (often to develop knowledge and skills in relation to a particular child's needs) and occasional placements. On their return, staff were then expected to share their learning with other staff.

Professionals' relationships with hospice staff

The professionals we interviewed (for example, health visitors, social workers, nurses) had varied experiences in terms of their relationships with the hospice. About a third of them had an 'easy' relationship with the hospice staff and tended to visit both formally and informally. Others found communication less straightforward:

> 'Communication with the hospice is an issue . . . they may be good at communicating with the families but they are reluctant to communicate with fellow professionals – usually on the basis of confidentiality.'

Two professionals observed that the hospice did not always involve them sufficiently in discussions or decisions regarding the care of a child they had referred – only being called in when there was a crisis or a major change in the service provided. They clearly felt excluded at times and uneasy about their relationship with the hospice staff. As one person observed:

> 'They have no "policy" on communicating with other professionals and tend to "take over", even though some people may have been working with the family for a number of years.'

Finally, for some professionals, it was the informality of the hospices which could be problematic. As one health professional commented:

> 'I have a problem with never knowing who you are talking to at the hospice. You don't know whether they are a qualified nurse or not [and] I feel this is something you need to know because you gear your approach accordingly.'

Volunteers

Hospices varied in the extent to which they recruited volunteers and how they used them. These volunteers were undertaking a wide range of tasks and their contributions were seen as important in lightening the load on paid staff. Observers noticed this during a visit to one hospice:

> At this particular session there were no volunteers, which left the [care] staff having to be responsible for the meal and clearing up after it. It was a demanding mix of children plus [there were] a number of parents and children who each had their own particular needs.

[On the following day] the addition of four volunteers enabled the staff to concentrate solely on the needs of the children, making for a more relaxed atmosphere.

Some volunteers undertook activities outside the hospice and were involved in:

- working (in pairs) in families' own homes either with the disabled child or with siblings;
- fund-raising for the hospice.

In the hospices, volunteers were involved in:

- gardening and general maintenance;
- cooking;
- cleaning;
- hydrotherapy pool attendants;
- driving;
- staffing the reception area.

Other volunteers worked directly with the children:

- stimulating them through play;
- helping them with eating.

Staff emphasised the importance of respecting the volunteers' contribution. As one volunteer coordinator said:

'They need to be respected in the sense that they work alongside professionals. They need to be treated as if they have intelligence . . . they need to be given confidence and information.'

Support for volunteers was also considered important and coordinators mentioned the need to support volunteers, while maintaining appropriate confidentiality:

'A lot of [volunteers] get very involved with the parents and they do need to talk to staff quite a lot . . . they need to be able to talk to each other as well about families they know although we do stress confidentiality.'

Formal supervision arrangements for volunteers varied between hospices and depended on the kind of tasks being undertaken. In one hospice, where volunteers were working one-to-one with children, there was no specific supervision but volunteers could always ask a member of staff for help. In the same hospice, where pairs of volunteers were doing 'outreach' work with families, there were monthly support meetings. These meetings, combined with the fact that volunteers were working in pairs, were seen as a sufficient means of providing support and monitoring the service provided, unless a home situation changed significantly.

Although the need for support was generally recognised, some staff who were interviewed implied that volunteers did not require supervision as such:

'The cleaners . . . we've had most of them since we started the volunteer scheme – they know more than we do.'

Volunteers were seen not only as a vital resource, but also as highly experienced in working with children and families.

Case study 7: John

John is 12 and lives with his mum, step-dad, and three-year-old sister, Jo. John's older brother, Craig, who had the same condition as John, died two years ago and John's dad died in a road accident when John was just a few months old.

The family live in a small market town. His step-dad works full time and his mum works part time when Jo is at the nearby childminder's. The ground floor of the family's house was adapted to enable both Craig and John to have their own space, so they can accommodate John's increasing needs for care and supervision.

John has Sanfillipo syndrome, a progressive disease which means he has learning difficulties and heart problems. His mum describes him as a lively boy with a 'wicked smile and a really good sense of humour' although his personality has changed and he does show increasingly difficult behaviour as his condition deteriorates.

Because Craig was also cared for at the hospice, the family feel they know the staff really well and they particularly appreciated the way they spent extra time with John when his brother died. 'John gets on really well with the hospice staff and they are good with him', his parents comment.

On a number of occasions, the whole family have stayed at the hospice and they feel quite at home there – though John's step-dad gets a bit bored when there aren't any other fathers staying!

John goes to a special school eight miles away and can still get there when he's staying at the hospice. Although his condition is deteriorating and he needs a lot more support, his mum feels it's important that he still goes to school while he can. He enjoys being round other children and, when he's well enough, enjoys going on school trips and being outdoors.

Once a month John stays overnight with another family. Having also offered breaks for Craig, they know, John's family well and are keen to continue offering their support for as long as they are able. Together with the hospice, John's mum feels this is just about enough to keep them ticking over.

7 Regulatory concerns

Introduction

The Children Act 1989 heralded a landmark in child care history, bringing disabled children within the same legal framework as other groups of children in need. Disabled children would have the same safeguards as other children, regardless of whether they were living with their families or elsewhere.

Unlike children's homes or foster placements, however, children's hospices were not included in the regulations, possibly because when the Act was introduced, few such places were in existence, but also because the government at that time had adopted a broadly non-interventionist stance in relation to voluntary bodies (particularly if they were not funded from the public purse).

With a change of government in 1997, however, there has been a growing concern about 'vulnerable' citizens – whether children or adults – and an increasing awareness of the need to develop frameworks which lessen the likelihood of abuse or neglect. The White Paper, *Modernising Social Services* (Department of Health, 1998) proposes a new framework for regulating both adults and children's services which attempts to reduce inconsistencies and promote greater coherence. Many of these proposals are welcome in the light of concerns raised by this research.

Registration and inspection

Children's hospices are currently registered as nursing homes by the local health authority, which means they are inspected at least twice a year, one of the visits being unannounced. Although this offers some safeguards, it has a number of shortcomings:

- the criteria are too general;
- issues such as safety are overemphasised at the expense of other concerns about the quality of care provided such as staff–child interactions;
- there is insufficient focus on issues relating specifically to children;
- inspection criteria do not allow for the fact that hospices are seeking to provide care in a homely, family-style environment.

However some hospices have found inspection officers to be accommodating and have been able to work with them in a more 'hospice-focused' way:

> '[Inspection is] workable . . . we have a very reasonable registra-tion officer . . . we have used the experience of [another children's hospice] and we have had a lot of help and support from them.'

The White Paper (see above) proposes a regulatory frame-work which would remove the distinction between nursing and residential care homes, and replace them with integrated national standards for nursing and social care. These will apply to *all* residential settings, whether private, voluntary or statutory. The maintenance of these standards will be dependent upon inspection which will be carried out by regional branches of the newly formed Commission for Care Standards (CCS).

The placement of individual children

The Children Act recognises that the child's welfare is paramount and the associated regulations, including those relating to children accommodated outside the family home, reflect this. Regulations (which could be) relevant to hospice care are as follows:

Section 22(4), 61 and 64 of the Children Act which require the ascertainable wishes and feelings of the child, and those of the parents and others with responsible authority, to be sought and taken into account before the individual plan is agreed.

The Children (Short Term Placements) (Miscellaneous Amendment) Regulations, 1995, 5(2) stipulate that the child's plan should be reviewed and amended regularly, but not less than three months after the child's first stay and subsequently at six-monthly intervals.

If these Children Act regulations were to apply to children's hospices, a social worker would have to be involved with each child (and family). This is not presently the case; indeed, some children and their families have never had a social worker. Even with those who do have one, contact may be discontinued once regular use of the hospice has been established, with families making their own arrangements directly with the hospice.

Perhaps because the Children Act regulations do not currently apply to children's hospices, regular meetings and reviews involving families are a comparatively rare event. Few families had been involved in a meeting to discuss their child's care at the hospice and only seven of the 17 professionals we interviewed said they were involved in regular meetings. Review meetings which did take place were generally held annually or bi-annually in order to consider whether the child's condition warranted continuing (use of) hospice care.

Although reviews of short-term placements under Children Act regulations have not always been particularly effective (Macadam and Robinson, 1995), they do offer a degree of protection to potentially vulnerable children and if introduced in hospices would:

- ensure that external professionals were involved and hospices had regular contact with social services;
- provide regular reviews of the suitability of a placement and an external professional would be responsible for finding an alternative placement if the hospice's services were not offered or were withdrawn;
- help counter the emphasis on 'health' by involving social services which provides a more 'holistic' approach and can consider a wider range of needs.

We welcome the proposal to introduce a more appropriate system of registration for all care homes and believe hospices are likely to benefit from a more integrated approach to all inspections.

At the same time, the *Arrangements for Placement of Children (General) Regulations 1991* and the *Review of Children's Cases Regulations 1991* should apply to children using hospices for short-term care.

Children's hospices, which are generally providing good quality care, may consider these changes unnecessary, but with the growth of the hospice movement it would seem appropriate to bring them within the same regulatory framework as other services providing (short-term) care to children and young people in order to establish basic safeguards.

Case study 8: Robin

Robin is 16 and lives with his mum and dad and 12-year-old sister, Chloe, just outside a small village. Robin's dad is self-employed and works from home; his mum works part time at a local farm shop. Both parents drive the family's wheelchair accessible vehicle, making it relatively easy for Robin to get around.

Robin has Duchenne Muscular Dystrophy and now needs a lot of help with washing and dressing. Although he can usually feed himself and, according to his mum, 'will eat anything', he occasionally has difficulty swallowing so needs to have someone around to make sure that he doesn't choke. The house has been adapted 'as far as possible' and Robin gets around in a powered wheelchair which he drives very fast when there's sufficient space.

Robin is described by his mum and dad as 'very bright'. He and Chloe attend the local comprehensive where he is studying for GCSEs. Although Robin has missed a lot of schooling over the years, he still manages to exceed his parents' and his teacher's expectations.

Robin's parents are keen that he has a full and active life and several friends who he has known since he was very young often come over to Robin's house to listen to music or play computer games.

Robin started going to the hospice about seven years ago. His mum was suffering from a stress-related illness at that time and the local health visitor who had regular contact with the hospice suggested it might meet the family's needs.

Initially, Robin went to the hospice once or twice a year but he now goes four or five times, usually at weekends, and on his own as that is what he prefers because he can 'let his hair down' away from home. He has made friends with a couple of other teenage boys and the three are often there at the same time – 'heaven for Robin but hell for the staff' as Robin's mother says.

Although the future is uncertain for Robin, his parents hope he can continue going to the hospice. They feel confident about the care he receives and for Robin it is one of the few places spacious enough for him to be independent once he's in his chair.

8 Recommendations for policy and practice

1 The role of the hospices

Children's hospices are faced with striking a difficult balance between providing a normal atmosphere and daily routine for children receiving short-term care, alongside the provision of intensive and sensitive care to very ill and dying children and their families. Given the relatively small number of children dying in hospices and the increasing emphasis on domicillary-based support for terminally ill children and their families, specialist terminal care units are not likely to be viable or, indeed, necessary.

1.1 Children's hospices should continue to fulfil a dual role, providing short-term care for children with life-limiting or life-threatening conditions as well as offering terminal and palliative care. However, this needs careful planning (see below).

1.2 Literature and other publicity should state explicitly that children's hospices mainly provide breaks for severely disabled children, although they may also provide palliative and terminal care.

1.3 Short-term care should be available to families on a planned and regular basis, but hospices should also continue to provide for emergency admissions.

1.4 Children's hospices should be planned and developed in conjunction with other services for children with high support needs and their families so that hospice care is part of a coordinated range of provision.

1.5 Hospice buildings should be designed to provide separate areas for children who are seriously and/or terminally ill (and their families).

2 The children's care

Hospices seek to provide high quality child-centred care, usually for a very diverse group, including: very young children through to adolescents and young adults; children who are very frail as well as those who are very physically active and who may exhibit challenging behaviour; and children from diverse ethnic and religious backgrounds. Activities need to be simulating and enjoyable and, during term-time, will often have to substitute for schooling.

2.1 The care offered in hospices should be appropriate for the individual children using the service in terms of their age, degree of disability and ethnic background.

2.2 Hospices should continue to cater for frail and non-mobile children as well as physically active children, but living and sleeping areas should be organised to accommodate these two groups separately where necessary.

2.3 Hospices must pay attention to developing more structured educational and play activities, ensuring a stimulating and enjoyable environment.

2.4 Special attention needs to be paid to the provision of activities and stimulation for children who have little or no verbal communication and/or multiple impairments and require assistance in order to participate in any organised activities.

2.5 Local education authorities should support the provision of peripatetic teaching staff for children using the hospice during term-time who are unable to attend their usual school.

2.6 Hospices need to carefully monitor for the potentially harmful effects of separating children from their families, and do what is necessary to minimise any immediate and longer-term distress.

2.7 Where a child is clearly distressed, staff should set up a review meeting with the family and relevant professionals to consider the use of alternative support.

2.8 To help provide continuity of care, each child should have a named person (or keyworker) who should help that child settle in and ensure that specific individual needs are being met appropriately.

2.9 Wherever possible, hospices should provide a keyworker who speaks the same language as the child and family.

2.10 Hospices will continue to cater for a mix of children, but should also consider offering special weeks to cater for particular groups, such as 'toddler breaks' or 'teenagers weeks'.

Services for young adults

2.11 Urgent consideration should be given to developing pilot schemes for young adults with neuro-muscular disorders requiring short breaks but for whom hospice care is no longer available. Local residential units, offering a degree of privacy and autonomy with on-call personal assistance, could also be a stepping-stone to supported/independent living.

3 Staffing and volunteers

Staff are the hospices' most important resource, often caring for children whose needs cannot be met (or only partially) by other local services. This care can be extremely taxing (particularly when terminally ill children are being looked after alongside other children), and effective supervision, support and ongoing training and development are essential to the provision of a quality service.

3.1 Staffing levels should reflect the numbers and needs of children using the hospice at any one time and additional staff should be available at short notice when necessary, which may necessitate employing a limited number of people on a retainer basis.

3.2 All hospice staff should receive regular supervision and support as well as having access to opportunities for ongoing training and development.

3.3 Staff training and development programmes should include cultural awareness training and assist staff in delivering a service which is sensitive to the cultural and religious practices of the children and families who use the hospice.

3.4 Particular attention should be paid to the support needs of staff providing terminal care.

3.5 Hospices should consider appointing staff with education experience to provide programmes of activities for the children and training and support for care staff.

3.6   Although the majority of hospice admissions are for short-term care, all staff should be trained to provide care for terminally ill children and their families.

3.7   Where the hospice catchment area includes significant minority ethnic communities, staff from these communities should be recruited, particularly where English is not the first language of the children and their families.

3.8   Hospices will need to implement the European Working Time Directive in ways which safeguard the interests of staff but which enable them to deliver a child-centred service in terms of providing continuity of care.

3.9   Volunteers whose activities involve unsupervised access to children should be subject to the same scrutiny as employees.

4 Access to hospices

Despite the fact that the number of children's hospices is growing steadily, the level of provision in some areas is not sufficient to meet demand and it is therefore particularly important that hospices actively target their services at those most in need.

4.1   When deciding whether to offer a service to a family, hospices should take account of factors such as the family's socio-economic circumstances as well as the child's level of disability and support needs.

4.2   Hospices which serve a large catchment area should urgently consider developing outreach services in addition to their buildings-based provision. This is particularly important for very young children.

4.3   Hospices serving areas with sizeable minority ethnic communities should be proactive in making hospice care available to families from these communities, by establishing contact with relevant local and community organisations and professionals.

5 Hospices and other services/professionals

Children's hospices have tended to develop largely in isolation from other short-term care services for children with disabilities. Much closer liaison is needed between hospice staff and local agencies both at a strategic level and in coordinating provision received by individual families.

5.1 Future hospice developments should be planned in conjunction with health and social services so that provision is seen as part of a coherent strategy for the care and support of children with life-threatening or life-limiting conditions and their families.

5.2 Hospices need to develop effective working relationships with other short-term care providers, and should be represented on local short-term care panels so that hospice care is an integrated part of a range of local provision.

5.3 Health and social services, together with the hospices, need to pool their knowledge and expertise, to develop non-residential supports to children with complex health needs and their families. Each agency can contribute to this learning. This could be particularly helpful in developing services to babies and young children for whom hospice care is not especially appropriate.

5.4 Closer liaison is needed between professionals support- ing families using hospices and the hospice staff so that families receive a coordinated package of support.

5.5 More active inter-agency working could also address the issue of transition to adult services for young people whose families may have difficulty accessing adult short-term care provision when they reach the upper age limit for hospice care.

6 Families

For many families, the hospice was a lifeline and their main or sole provider of breaks. However, communication between hospice staff and families was often limited to contact at the beginning and end of a child's stay. Although the availability of family accommodation is appreciated by families, particu- larly when a child is new to a hospice or is ill, in practice only a small number of families used it.

6.1 Families should meet with hospice staff, including their child's keyworker, at least twice a year so that they are kept informed about any changes in the hospice service

but also so that they can discuss their child's care while
there.

6.2 All hospices should strive to provide good quality family
accommodation although this should not be on a large
scale as demand is likely to continue to be limited.

7 Funding

Children's hospices are filling an important gap in current
provision and as more severely disabled children survive
beyond the first days or months, demand for services is likely
to increase. However, they usually rely heavily on charitable
fund-raising, receiving only limited finance from NHS trusts
or local authorities.

7.1 Central government should issue guidance on the
future funding of children's hospices.

7.2 Health and social services should be encouraged to use
their pooled budgets to finance additional short-term
care for severely disabled children with healthcare
needs.

7.3 Families should not be expected to meet the costs of
hospice care themselves, given the additional costs of
caring for a severely disabled child.

8 Regulation

There are two main areas of regulatory concern: statutory
registration and inspection of children's hospices; and
arrangements for monitoring and reviewing the placement
of individual children, including the suitability of hospice care
and the quality of care provided.

8.1 Placement of individual children in hospice care should
be carried out in accordance with the Children Act to
ensure that external professionals are involved in all
placements and that those placements are regularly
reviewed by the hospice, the family and relevant
professionals.

8.2 Regulation and inspection of children's hospices, together with arrangements for placement of individual
children, should be consistent with the spirit and

intention of the Children Act 1989, ensuring that disabled children are within the same regulatory framework as other 'children in need'.

8.3 Children hospices should be regulated by the independent, statutory regional Commissions for Care Standards proposed in the recent White Paper, *Modernising Social Services* (1998).

8.4 Hospices should implement the recommendations of the Government's response to the Children's Safeguards Review (1998), including the development of an accessible complaints procedure, use of the Consultancy Service Index and promotion of children's involvement in planning for their care.

Appendix

Table A1   The average age of children in each hospice

Hospice	Mean age
Aster House	2 years 2 months
Begonia House	9 years 9 months
Cherry Blossoms	10 years 8 months
Daisy Way	10 years 8 months
All hospices	9 years 7 months

Table A2   Diagnoses

Diagnosis category*	Number	%
Diseases of the nervous system, e.g. cerebral palsy (n=63) and muscular dystrophy (n=59)	188	52.5
Congenital abnormalities including: (a) reduction deficiencies of the brain such as microcephaly (n=38) (b) other and unspecified abnormalities such as Tuberous Sclerosis and Rubenstein Taybi syndrome (n=33) (c) chromosonal abnormalities, e.g. Down's and Patau's syndrome (n=18)	106	29.6
Endocrine, nutritional and metabolic diseases	26	7.3
Neoplasms	14	3.9
No diagnosis	7	2.0
Diseases of the genito-urinary system and chronic renal failure	6	1.7
Diseases of the circulatory system	4	1.1
Diseases of blood and bloodforming organs	2	0.6
Mental disorders	2	0.6
Diseases of the digestive system	2	0.6
Head injury – non accidental	1	0.3

*For an explanation of these categories, please refer to International Classification of Disease (ICD) 9

Table A3   Nursing interventions

Type of nursing care	Number of children*	% of children
Administration of drugs	270	75.4
Feeding via gastrostomy tube	70	19.6
Suction	55	15.4
Enemas or suppositories	40	11.2
Feeding via naso-gastric tube	39	10.9
Nebulliser	31	8.6
Administration of rectal diazepam	29	8.1
Administration of oxygen	29	8.1
Replacement of dressings	20	5.6
Tracheostomy	13	3.6
Catheter care	13	3.6
Splints/brace	6	1.7
Injections	5	1.4
Syringe driven pump	5	1.4
Dialysis	4	1.1
Ieostomy or colostomy	4	1.1
Central venous pressure line	4	1.1
Blood tests	2	0.5
Oral hygiene	2	0.5
Observation of vital signs	2	.5

*Not cumulative as children could have up to five 'nursing interventions'

Table A4   The range of drug types prescribed to children

Medication	Number of times type of drugs cited*	Number of children*	% of children
Anti-epileptics	297	179	50.0
Laxatives	132	93	26.0
Bronchodilators, inhalers	97	57	15.9
Analgesics	89	82	22.9
Anti-spasmodics and acid inhibitors	76	60	16.8
Antibiotics	72	67	18.7
Sedatives	57	52	14.5
Hypnotics and antidepressants	39	37	10.3
Vitamins	32	26	7.3
Drugs for muscular spasms	32	30	8.4
Iron/folic acid	20	17	4.7
Cough mixtures/nasal decongestant preparations	18	17	4.7

Table A4   *continued*

Medication	Number of times type of drugs cited*	Number of children*	% of children
Drugs for nausea and vertigo	17	16	4.5
Skin creams	17	16	4.5
Anti-inflammatories including topical preparations	16	14	3.9
Minerals and electrolytes	16	13	3.6
Antidiarrhoeals	15	15	4.2
Corticosteroids	14	13	3.6
Antihistamines	11	11	3.1
Oral rehydration	11	11	3.1
Antihypertensives	10	8	2.2
Food supplements	10	7	2.0
Eye drops	9	9	2.5
Drugs for genito-urinary conditions	8	6	1.7
Diuretics	7	7	2.0
Supplements for metabolic disorders	6	5	1.4
Oral hygiene/drugs acting on oropharynx	6	5	1.4
Growth hormones	4	4	1.1
Anticoagulants	3		0.8
Oxygen	3	3	0.8
Insulin	3	3	0.8
Gout treatments	3	3	0.8
Antibacterial skin preparations	3	3	0.8
Inotropic drugs	2	2	0.6
Drugs affecting intestinal secretions	2	1	0.3
Antimuscarin drugs	2	2	0.6
Immuno modulators	2	2	0.6
Ear drops	2	2	0.6
Thyroid treatments	1	1	0.3
Anti-protozoal	1	1	0.3
Anaesthetics	1	1	0.3

*Not cumulative

Table A5   Parents' expectations of hospices

Parents' expectations of hospices	Number (n=38)*	% of chidren
Frequent breaks	18	47.4
Good professional care	8	28.6
Emergency care	6	15.8
A flexible package	6	15.8
One-to-one care	6	15.8
24 hour cover	5	13.2
A break from the routine of caring	4	10.5
They will cater for a wide range of needs	3	7.9
Time-limited care	3	7.9
Infrequent breaks at first	2	5.3
Care for all the family	2	5.3
A place for children to die	2	5.3
More help than before	2	5.3
Not a well resourced environment	1	2.6
A good rapport with the staff	1	2.6
The child had to be in a cot	1	2.6
Nothing or not clear expectations	5	13.2

*Not cumulative as parents could have more than one expectation

Bibliography

ACT (1994) *The ACT Charter for children with life-threatening conditions and their families.* Association for Children with Life-Threatening or Terminal Conditions and their Families

ACT and the Royal College of Paediatrics and Child Health (1997) *Children's Palliative Care Services.* Report of a joint working party. Association for Children with Life-Threatening or Terminal Conditions and their Families, and the Royal College of Paediatrics and Child Health

Association of Children's Hospices (ACH) (1995) *Guidelines for Good Practice in a Children's Hospice.* Association of Children's Hospices

Avebury, K (1984) *Home Life: a code of practice for residential care.* Report of a Working Party sponsored by the DHSS and convened by the Centre for Policy on ageing under the Chairmanship of Kina, Lady Avebury

Baldwin, S (1985) *The Costs of Caring.* Routledge and Kegan Paul

Baum, J D, Dominica, F and Woodward, R N eds (1990) *"Listen my child has a lot of living to do". Caring for children with life-threatening conditions.* Oxford University Press

Baxter, C, Poonia, K, Ward, L and Nadirshaw, Z (1990) *Double Discrimination.* Kings Fund Centre/Commission for Racial Equality

Bercusson, B (1994) *Working in Time in Britain: Towards a European Model. Part 1: The European Union Directive.* Institute of Employment Rights

Burne, R, Baum, D and Dominica, F (1984*)* 'Helen House – a hospice for children: analysis of the first year', *British Medical Journal*, 289, 1665–68

Campbell, A G M and McIntosh, N eds (1992) *Forfar and O'Neill's Textbook of Paediatrics*, 4th edn. Churchill Livingstone

Carlisle, D (1988) 'From hospice to respite', *Nursing Standard*, 2, 45, 20

Carroll, L and Reilly, S (1996) 'The therapeutic approach to the child with feeding difficulty: management and treatment' *in* Sullivan, P and Rosenbloom, L eds *Feeding the Disabled Child.* MacKeith Press

Chadwick, H (1993) 'A comparison of general practitioners' and parents' perceptions of a children's hospice.' Masters thesis, Social Work Department, University of Southampton

Chambers, T L (1987) 'Hospices for Children?' (Editorial) *British Medical Journal*, 294 (6583), 1309

Clarke, D ed. (1993a) *The Future for Palliative Care: Issues of Policy and Practice*. Open University Press

Clarke, D (1993b) 'Whither Hospices?' *in* Clarke, D ed. *The Future for Palliative Care: Issues of Policy and Practice*. Open University Press.

Clayden, G and Hawkins, R eds (1988) *Paediatrics*. Heinemann Medical

Contact A Family (1997) *The CAF Directory of Specific Conditions and Rare Syndromes in Children with their Family Support Networks*. Contact A Family

Department of Health (1996) *The Regulation and Inspection of Social Services*. Report by Tom Burgner. The Stationery Office

Department of Health (1997a) *Children's Homes at 31st March 1997, England*. Department of Health

Department of Health (1997b) *The New NHS, Modern, Dependable* (White Paper). The Stationery Office

Department of Health (1998) *Modernising Social Services* (White Paper). The Stationery Office

Gordon, D, Parker, R and Loughran, F (1996) *Children with disabilities in Private Households: A Re-analysis of the Office of Population Censuses and Surveys' Investigation*. Report to the Department of Health. School of Policy Studies, University of Bristol

Green, J M and Murton, F E (1993) *Duchenne Muscular Dystrophy: The experiences of 158 families*. Centre for Family Research, University of Cambridge.

Hathaway, W E et al. eds (1990) *Current Paediatric Diagnosis and Treatment*, 14, p. 1139. Norwalk, Conneticut: Appleton & Lange

Herd, E (1990) 'Helen House' *in* Baum, J D, Dominica, F and Woodward, R N eds *"Listen my child has a lot of living to do". Caring for children with life-threatening conditions*. Oxford University Press

Hochstadt, N J and Yost, D M eds (1991) *The Medically Complex Child. The Transition to Home*. Philadelphia, USA: Harwood Academic Publishers

Hutchinson, T (1997) Personal communication, concerning the numbers of disabled children receiving suction

Kagan, C, Lewis, S and Heaton, P (1998) *Caring to Work: Accounts of working parents of disabled children*. Family Policy Studies Centre

Kohrman, A F (1992) 'Implications of medical technology' *in* Hochstadt, N J and Yost, D M eds *The Medically Complex Child. The Transition to Home*. Philadelphia, USA: Harwood Academic Publishers

Lenehan, C (1989) *Respite Care in the East End: a multicultural challenge*. Barnardos

Macadam, M and Robinson, C (1995) *Balancing the Act. The Impact of the Children Act 1989 on family link services for children with disabilities*. National Children's Bureau

Martin House (1994) Personal communication with Carol Robinson, about the numbers of children accommodated for short-term care

Meltzer, H, Smyth, M and Robus, N (1989) *Disabled children: services, transport and education*. OPCS surveys of disability in Great Britain, Report 6. HMSO

Micklewright, A (1996) 'Experience of long-term home enteral nutrition in Europe: United Kingdom.' Paper presented to the XVIII Espen Congress, 8–11 September 1996, Geneva

Minkes, J, Robinson, C and Weston, C (1994) 'Consulting the children: interviews with children using residential respite care services', *Disability & Society*, 9, 1

Morris, J (1998) *Still Missing? The experiences of disabled children and young people living away from their families*. Volume 1. Who Cares? Trust

Nash, T (1998) *The needs of families with children suffering from life limiting or threatening illnesses in the South West: Summary of findings*. University of Exeter, Department of Sociology

Newitt, B, Jones, V and Robinson, C (1998) *Quality Counts. A Review of quality assurance in family based short term care*. Shared Care UK

Oswin, M (1984) *They Keep Going Away. A critical study of short-term residential care services for children who are mentally handicapped*. Kings Fund and Oxford University Press

Powell, T H and Gallagher, P A (1993) *Brothers and Sisters – A special part of exceptional families*. Baltimore, USA: Paul H Brookes Publishing Co

Quine, L and Pahl, J (1989) *Stress and coping in families caring for a child with severe mental handicap: A longitudinal Survey*. University of Kings, Canterbury: Institute of Social and Applied Psychology and Centre for Health Services Studies

Rendle-Short, J, Gray, O P and Dodge, J A eds (1985) *A Synopsis of Children's Diseases*. 6th edn. Wright

Rhodes, A, Lenehan, C and Morrison, J (1998) *Supporting Children who need invasive clinical procedures: A guide for Barnardo's family support services*. Barnardos

Robinson, C (1986) *Avon Short Term Respite Care Scheme. Evaluation. Volumes 1 and 2*. Norah Fry Research Centre, University of Bristol

Robinson, C and Stalker, K (1989) *Time for a Break. Respite Care: A Study of Providers, Consumers and Patterns of Use*. First Interim report to the Department of Health. Norah Fry Research Centre, University of Bristol

Robinson, C and Stalker, K (1990) *Respite care – the Consumer's View. Second Interim report to the Department of Health*. Norah Fry Research Centre, University of Bristol

Robinson, C, Weston, C and Minkes, J (1996) *Quality in Residential Short Term Care Services*. The Stationery Office

Salvage, J (1986) *Hospices for children: a need in a sick society?* Proceedings of a conference organised jointly by the King's Fund Centre and Helen House Hospice for Children, held at the King's Fund Centre, 2 December 1986. KF No. 86/181, King's Fund Centre, London

Servian, R, Jones, V, Lenehan, C and Spires, S (1998) *Towards a Healthy Future: Multiagency working in the management of invasive and life-saving procedures for children in family based services*. Policy Press for Shared Care Network

Stalker, K and Robinson, C (1994) 'Parents' views of different respite care services', *Mental Handicap Research*, 7, 2, 97–117

Stein, A and Woolley, H (1990) 'An evaluation of hospice care for children' *in* Baum, J D, Dominica, F and Woodward, R N *eds* "*Listen my child has a lot of living to do*". *Caring for children with life-threatening conditions*. Oxford University Press

Thompson, R J and O'Quinn, A N (1979) *Developmental disabilities: aetiologies, manifestations and treatments*. New York: Oxford University Press

Thornes, R (1990) 'Towards a comprehensive system of care for dying children and their families: key issues' *in* Baum, J D, Dominica, F and Woodward, R N *eds* "*Listen my child has a lot of living to do*". *Caring for children with life-threatening conditions*. Oxford University Press

Townsley, R and Robinson, C (1997a) *On Line Support. Effective services to disabled children who are tube fed*. Interim report to NHS Executive. Norah Fry Research Centre, University of Bristol

Townsley, R and Robinson, C (1997b) 'Comfort Eating', *Nursing Times*, 93, 34, August 1997, Nutrition Supplement

Utting, W, Baines, C, Stuart, M *et al.* (1997) *People like us: The report of the review of the safeguards for children living away from home*. The Stationery Office

Wagner, G (1988) *A positive Choice. Report of the Independent Review of Residential Care, chaired by Gillian Wagner*. National Institute for Social Work

While, A, Citrone, C and Cornish, J (1996) *A study of the needs and provisions for families caring for children with life-limiting incurable disorders*. Department of Nursing Studies, Kings College, London

World Health Organisation (WHO) (1975) *Manual of International Statistical Classification of Diseases and Injuries and Causes of Death, 1 & 2*. Geneva: WHO

Acts and Regulations

Children Act 1989

Arrangements for Placement of Children (General) Regulations, 1991

Children's Homes Regulations, 1991

Department of Health (1991) *Review of Children's Cases Regulations*

The Children (Short Term Placements) (Miscellaneous Amendments) Regulations, 1995

Index